Fight Diabetes
with Vitamins and
Antioxidants

"Dr. Prasad, a leading investigator and advocate for the role of micronutrients in cancer and neurodegenerative disorders, now succinctly presents an excellent biological rationale for the use of vitamins and antioxidants in the prevention and treatment of diabetes. His biological perspectives of micronutrients and concise meta-analysis of the existing data can help readers to consider antioxidants and proper agents in the fight against chronic disorders, especially for diabetes and cancer."

JAE HO KIM, M.D., PH.D., PROFESSOR OF RADIATION ONCOLOGY,
HENRY FORD HEALTH SYSTEM, DETROIT, MICHIGAN

"This is a most insightful presentation with many key ideas concerning both the prevention of onset and the deterrence of progression of diabetes. In view of the explosive increase in incidence of this disease, this book is especially timely. Emphasis is placed on inexpensive and noninvasive means by which diabetes patients can take command of a significant portion of their treatment. This makes the book especially valuable and relevant to a wide readership."

STEPHEN C. BONDY, PH.D., PROFESSOR, CENTER FOR
OCCUPATIONAL AND ENVIRONMENTAL HEALTH, DEPARTMENT OF
MEDICINE, UNIVERSITY OF CALIFORNIA, IRVINE

Fight Diabetes

with Vitamins and Antioxidants

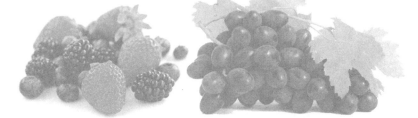

Kedar N. Prasad, Ph.D.

Healing Arts Press
Rochester, Vermont • Toronto, Canada

Healing Arts Press
One Park Street
Rochester, Vermont 05767
www.HealingArtsPress.com

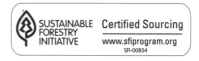

Text stock is SFI certified

Healing Arts Press is a division of Inner Traditions International

*Note to the reader: This book is intended as an informational guide. The remedies,
approaches, and techniques described herein are meant to supplement, and not to be a
substitute for, professional medical care or treatment. They should not be used to treat
a serious ailment without prior consultation with a qualified health care professional.*

Library of Congress Cataloging-in-Publication Data
Prasad, Kedar N.
  Fight diabetes with vitamins and antioxidants / Kedar N. Prasad, Ph.D.
     pages cm
  Includes bibliographical references and index.
  ISBN 978-1-62055-166-0 (pbk.) — ISBN 978-1-62055-172-1 (e-book)
  1. Diabetes—Alternative treatment. 2. Diabetes—Nutritional aspects. 3. Vitamin
therapy. 4. Orthomolecular therapy. I. Title.
  RC661.A47P73 2014
  616.4'62061—dc23

                                                              2013032985

Printed and bound in the United States by Lake Book Manufacturing, Inc.
The text stock is SFI certified. The Sustainable Forestry Initiative® program
promotes sustainable forest management.

10 9 8 7 6 5 4 3 2 1

Text design and layout by Virginia Scott Bowman
This book was typeset in Garamond Premier Pro and Gill Sans with Helvetica and
Gill Sans used as the display typefaces

To send correspondence to the author of this book, mail a first-class letter to the
author c/o Inner Traditions • Bear & Company, One Park Street, Rochester, VT
05767, and we will forward the communication, or contact the author directly at
kprasad@mypmcinside.com.

Contents

ACKNOWLEDGMENTS

I thank K. Che Prasad, M.S., M.D., for editing this work and for making very valuable suggestions.

Foreword

James Ehrlich, M.D.

I am a clinical advisor for Premier Micronutrient Corporation, a company formed to develop healthy products based upon the research efforts of a team of radiation biologists and micronutrient scientists led by Dr. Kedar N. Prasad. As a clinical associate professor in endocrinology whose major research has involved diabetics, I have had the privilege to witness the far-reaching activities of Dr. Prasad, a longtime professor at the University of Colorado, and the director for the Center for Vitamins and Cancer Research. I have always admired his teaching abilities, his honest research, and his leadership and passion for making a difference in the lives of individuals suffering from a great variety of disorders. He has published over two hundred papers, contributed chapters to many books, and authored or edited eighteen books of his own on the subjects of radiobiology, nutrition, and cancer.

For over three decades, Dr. Prasad has been remarkably convincing in promoting an underappreciated central thesis, one which I believe can greatly improve the health of millions of people the world over. He has consistently advocated the value of a scientifically based, multiple antioxidant approach to oxidative-stress-related disorders. This approach takes into consideration the disease state, kinetics (time-course) of therapy, efficacious tissue levels of micronutrients, and potential interactions with adjuvants (e.g., heavy metals). I have reviewed the protocols of many widely cited studies involving micronutrients as they relate to vascular disease, and I only wish that the authors of those studies had employed Dr. Prasad when constructing their study designs. The conclusions of a few of these fatally flawed contemporary studies might be quite different if they had done so!

Over the past several years there has been growing evidence that oxidative stress and inflammation are contributing factors to the development of various cardiometabolic disorders. In this, it has become increasingly clear that free radicals play an important role in the etiology and pathogenesis of diabetes and its complications. Contemporary research in vascular biology and diabetes has contributed to a better understanding of the link between oxidative stress and inflammation, and diabetic vascular complications and the progression of disease.

Much of this research has been focused on the generation of advanced glycation end-products: the result of non-enzymatic glycation and the oxidation of lipids and proteins. The deleterious effect of these by-products of metabolism on vascular beds and organs in patients with diabetes is an emerging area of intense activity, which has prompted a search for novel therapies that might disrupt the generation of such toxic species.

To compound these harmful effects, metabolic stress and tissue damage in diabetic patients can amplify oxidative damage, leading to a free-radical burden that can overwhelm natural scavenger mechanisms. In addition, atherogenic-oxidized lipoproteins, a by-product of diabetes, is a strong contributor to atherosclerosis and its progression in these patients. And with its dangerous partner in crime—inflammation—a cascade of life-threatening events can be set in motion. This frequently begins with unstable plaque, which too often leads to coronary and peripheral vascular disease, stroke, kidney failure, and sudden death.

If it is true that substantial research has already addressed these issues, why does the nation's preeminent micronutrient scientist/radiation biologist, Dr. Kedar N. Prasad, need to revisit them by writing this book? In my view, there are four pressing reasons:

1. **The *importance* of the subject due to the *magnitude* of the problem:** It is clear that diabetes and its increasingly prevalent precursor, metabolic syndrome, collectively represent *the* epidemic of the twenty-first century. The alarming and escalating magnitude of diabetes, given its spiraling health-related complications and expenses, makes it mandatory to reconsider better ways of managing and preventing the disease and its sequelae. That the disease is predominantly related to adverse trends in lifestyle and that it affords multiple targets of preventive therapy are factors that contribute to the vital importance of this subject.

2. **Knowledge gap:** As I have stated, our understanding of the relationship between diabetes and its complications that are derived from oxidative stress and inflammation is growing. However, this research has *not* filtered down to the practitioner in a measurable way that would require the practitioner to recommend additional risk-reduction strategies for patients afflicted with diabetes and metabolic syndrome. And without a clear understanding of the inherent properties of individual micronutrients and how they are best utilized in a multiple-antioxidant strategy, the consumer is left with a dizzying array of noxious, illogical therapies. Consequently, there is currently little chance that patients (including proactive citizens) will understand why and how to incorporate a micronutrient plan to minimize oxidative stress and inflammation in the potential mitigation of their disease.

3. **Misconceptions about vitamins and micronutrients:** The field of nutrition and the correct supplementation with proper micronutrients and vitamins has been extensively infiltrated by misconception and fallacy. With increasing frequency, practitioners are recommending—and vulnerable citizens are consuming—individual supplements, or combinations of supplements, which are unnecessary, ineffective, or downright damaging. In most cases, physicians do not address the nutritional

needs of their patients. This is due to a lack of interest and/or training, or because these physicians may not be reimbursed for nutritional counseling. Without authoritative guidebooks (such as those on vitamins and micronutrients that Dr. Prasad has been publishing for decades), or input from knowledgeable clinicians, these misconceptions are self-perpetuating ones that take on the veneer of scientific fact while promoting useless and/or even harmful therapies.

4. **The *need* for a *logical,* science-based *strategy* and a *call to action***: The research findings in the field of oxidative stress and diabetes have heretofore not been organized into a strategic therapeutic plan that can benefit patients afflicted with diabetes or those at risk for it. To motivate a change of behavior there needs to be a clear call to action by an authority who can debunk the misconceptions and translate scientific research into a comprehensive, logical, and practical clinical nutritional strategy.

In this book, Dr. Kedar N. Prasad brings decades of groundbreaking contributions to the micronutrient field to address all four of these critical needs in a compelling and scholarly manner. After setting the stage with a clear explanation of the scope of the modern epidemic of diabetes and its complications, he introduces the reader to the fundamental principles and pathophysiology of oxidative stress and inflammation. The complete mechanistic and measurable factors involved, the "cast of characters" if you will, include various detrimental contributors (cytokines, inflammatory particles, free radicals, etc.), important biomarkers, and laboratory assays for assessing oxidative stress and its effects. All are presented with extraordinary clarity and detail.

Next, Dr. Prasad systematically addresses the critical and prevalent knowledge gap that exists among patients and physicians alike while forthrightly debunking dangerous practices and misconceptions about the role and function of micronutrients in various clinical situations. In particular, potentially harmful and disturbingly common practices and poorly designed research protocols (e.g., using vitamin E alone, or combining vitamin C with certain metals) are challenged by Dr. Prasad in a convincing and logical fashion. Armed with the fundamental principles of addressing free radicals and inflammation, the clinician and diabetic patient are empowered to consider a targeted supplemental strategy that is likely to improve outcomes. This mandate to fight diabetes in a practical, safe, and logical manner, which complements all other proven recommendations and tactics for addressing the devastating disease, might be the most important benefit of this unique book.

As a colleague and admirer of the leadership that Dr. Prasad has displayed in research, teaching, and writing, I cannot imagine a more knowledgeable authority to create the book you now hold in your hands. I believe it will appeal to a great range of individuals—from the scientifically curious layperson to the proactive diabetic patient to the vascular biologist and, finally, to the health care practitioner and clinical nutritionist. If you are a clinician, I hope that *Fight Diabetes with Vitamins and Antioxidants* results in a re-examination of your clinical practice in such a way as to benefit your patients. If you are reading it because you are hoping to find help for your own diabetic disorder or because you want to prevent this disease from affecting others, please share this book with (or buy it as a valuable gift for) family and friends. It could very well represent the most important hidden weapon in our common, collective fight against this devastating disease.

DR. JAMES EHRLICH graduated with honors from Boston University School of Medicine in 1976. He attained his internship and residency training at the University of Colorado Health Sciences Center, where he remained as a clinical assistant professor in the Department of Anesthesiology, a specialty he practiced for twenty years. Dr. Ehrlich is the medical director and founder of Colorado Heart Imaging (CHI) in Denver, a preventive medical imaging facility that uses electron-beam tomography for the early detection of coronary disease and cancer. He is the medical co-director of similar facilities in Houston, Washington, D.C., and Boston, and consults for several other imaging centers nationally and in Europe. Dr. Ehrlich is currently on the staff of University Hospital and Rose Medical Center in Denver as well as being a clinical advisor for Premier Micronutrient Corporation.

Why Should You Read This Book?

Despite current preventative recommendations that involve changes in diet and lifestyle, the incidence of diabetes is increasing throughout the world, including in the United States. This implies that the proposed recommendations are not having the desired outcomes. If there are no significant changes in the current preventative recommendations for reducing the risk of this disease, it is estimated that by 2034 the number of people in the United States with diagnosed and undiagnosed diabetes will be approximately 44 million, up from roughly 23 million in 2009. The annual cost of this disease is currently $113 billion; it is expected to triple by 2034 (Huang et al. 2009).

The exact reasons for the failure of the current therapeutic approaches are difficult to ascertain with any degree of certainty. It is entirely possible that people are just not following the guidelines recommending changes in diet and lifestyle. Major diabetes-related complications such as retinopathy (damage to the eyes), nephropathy (damage to the kidneys), neuropathy (damage to the nervous system), and heart disease continue to develop, and at alarming rates, despite the use of current medications.

This is no doubt due to the fact that much of this medication is only designed to normalize plasma glucose levels. Increased oxidative stress and chronic inflammation, which play an important role in the development of diabetes and diabetes-related complications, are not influenced by these medications. Therefore, supplementation with antioxidants that serve to reduce oxidative stress and chronic inflammation would appear to be a logical choice in combatting this disease.

Although antioxidants and other agents acting together in synergistic fashion could be useful in reducing the risk of diabetes, they are not usually recommended by most doctors. This is due to the fact that many doctors believe that taking antioxidants may reduce the effectiveness of their therapy. However, this belief has no sound scientific basis because there are no conclusive data to support that an appropriate preparation of micronutrients containing multiple dietary and endogenous antioxidants can interfere with the effectiveness of current medications.

As regards research, only a *few* studies with individual antioxidants and omega-3 fatty acids (n-3 long-chain polyunsaturated fatty acids) have been performed, and *no* studies have been performed that evaluate the effectiveness of a micronutrient preparation containing multiple dietary and endogenous antioxidants, B vitamins, vitamin D, chromium picolinate, omega-3 fatty acids, and certain minerals, in combination with standard care.

This book clarifies the confusion about the value of antioxidants and other agents in reducing the risk of diabetes. It also provides scientific data to support the use of a preparation of micronutrients containing multiple dietary and endogenous antioxidants, B vitamins, vitamin D, and certain minerals in combination with changes in diet and lifestyle.

I hope it will serve as a guide for consumers in selecting an appropriate micronutrient preparation, and help people to make the changes that are necessary to reduce the risk of diabetes and improve its treatment outcomes. Consumers who are currently taking daily supplements will find the information in this book encouraging. Those who are not taking supplements or are uncertain about their potential benefit may find evidence to help them make a decision as to whether or not to take micronutrient supplements daily, in consultation with their doctors.

1 What Is Diabetes?

History, Causes, and Costs

The disease we call diabetes, also known as diabetes mellitus,* has existed throughout human history. Its earliest mention is found in the Ebers papyrus, an ancient Egyptian medical text dating to 1550 BCE. In the second century a disciple of Hippocrates by the name of Galen (130–210 CE) had knowledge of and discussed the disease but it was Aretaeus, Galen's contemporary, who coined the word "diabetes" and gave us the first true description of it. The ancient Hindus called diabetes "honey urine," and recorded how flies and ants were attracted to the urine of those persons afflicted with it (thus providing an early technique of diagnosis).

Diabetes mellitus is a disease marked by dysfunction as to how the body utilizes blood sugar, or glucose, which is the body's primary fuel. After the digestion of food, glucose enters the bloodstream where it is taken up by the cells of the body in order to maintain growth and provide energy. Insulin and glucagon, both made by the pancreas, are responsible for glucose uptake by the cells. If the pancreas is producing either insufficient amounts of insulin, or none at all, it is difficult for glucose to be used by the cells for generating energy. This results in increased levels of glucose in the blood—a condition known as

---

*Diabetes mellitus is distinguished from diabetes insipidus, a relatively rare disease that does not affect blood sugar levels but results in excessive urine production.

hyperglycemia. Diabetes is a chronic disease that is characterized by hyperglycemia, primarily due to insufficient or a total lack of insulin production by the pancreas, and/or as a result of the development of insulin resistance by the tissues of the body.

This chapter presents an overview of the different types of diabetes and the possible causes of them. We will also discuss its risk factors, conditions, and complications. Let's start by examining the three primary types of diabetes first.

TYPES OF DIABETES
AND THEIR COST TO SOCIETY

There are three major types of diabetes: type 1 diabetes, type 2 diabetes, and gestational diabetes (Cotran et al. 1999). Type 1 diabetes is inherited from one's parents as a genetic defect and is found primarily in children. In this type of diabetes, insulin production by the pancreas is insufficient due to the progressive death of insulin-producing cells. The ensuing hyperglycemia requires daily injections of insulin in order for normal blood glucose levels to be maintained.

In type 2 diabetes, sufficient amounts of insulin are initially produced by the pancreas but then a resistance to it develops, which causes hyperglycemia. Type 2 diabetes occurs mostly in young adults and adults and is considered an acquired disease, not an inherited one.

Gestational diabetes is a disease of pregnant women who develop it late in their pregnancy. It typically resolves of its own accord before the baby is born, but nevertheless has implications as regards type 2 susceptibility for the pregnant woman later on.

As people live longer, the management of chronic diseases, including diabetes, has become increasingly important. Despite current prevention and treatment strategies, the incidence of diabetes is rising. In the United States it is the seventh leading cause of death and the leading cause of kidney failure, blindness, and non-traumatic lower limb amputations. Having diabetes also increases one's risk of heart disease.

According to the 2011 National Diabetes Fact Sheet (the most current statistics available), the number of persons in the United States with diabetes equaled approximately 18.8 million individuals, with undiagnosed cases estimated to be approximately 7 million persons CDC Data & Trends, 2012 . People under the age of twenty with either type 1 or type 2 diabetes numbered approximately 215,000 individuals, and 79 million people were prediabetic. In 2010, newly diagnosed diabetics in persons older than twenty numbered 1.9 million, up from almost 500,000 in 1980. African Americans were the most impacted group (versus Latinos and Caucasians) and slightly more men than women were diagnosed with the disease. (Please see appendix I for a further articulation of these figures and trends.)

In terms of the future, it is estimated that between 2009 and 2034 the number of people with diagnosed and undiagnosed diabetes will increase from 23.7 million to 44.1 million, and about 65 percent of the general population will remain overweight or obese. In this same timeframe (2009–2034), it is estimated that the annual cost of managing diabetes will increase from $113 billion to $336 billion. For the Medicare-eligible population, the number of cases of diabetes is expected to increase from 8.2 million in 2009 to 14.6 million in 2034. The cost of managing diabetes in this population will increase from $45 billion to $171 billion (Huang et al. 2009). Medical costs for people with the disease are approximately two times higher than for those without it; these costs will continue to rise in future.

These projected expenses are astronomically high, causing one to wonder just how this disease has spiraled out of control. In order to understand the complexity of diabetes—its cost to society and its deleterious impact on individuals the world over—it is important to have a basic understanding of where it all begins: the human pancreas.

THE PANCREAS

A normal pancreas is responsible for producing and releasing insulin into the bloodstream. It is a pinkish-tan, elongated organ about 15 centimeters in length, located behind the stomach and close to the duodenum (part of the small intestine). Divided into three parts—head, body, and tail—it weighs 60–140 grams in an adult human being. The pancreas consists of two types of glands: the endocrine gland and the exocrine gland.

The Endocrine Gland

The endocrine gland contains approximately 1 million tiny clusters of cells (that can be seen only under the microscope), called the islets of Langerhans. In adults, islet cells contain four main types of cells as follows:

1. Alpha-cells (α-cells) produce glucagon, which raises blood glucose levels whenever they fall below the normal value.
2. Beta-cells (ß-cells) represent about 68 percent of the islet cell population and are responsible for producing insulin.
3. Delta-cells (δ-cells) produce somatostatin, which suppresses the release of both insulin and glucagon.
4. Pancreatic polypeptide cells (PP) contain a polypeptide that stimulates the secretion of gastric and intestinal enzymes and inhibits intestinal motility (movement).

The Exocrine Gland

The exocrine gland represents approximately 80–85 percent of the pancreas and contains numerous small glands called the acini. Every day the acinar glands secrete about 2 to 2.5 liters of bicarbonate-rich fluid, which contains digestive enzymes. These enzymes are released, in an inactive form, through a complex network of pancreatic ducts into the common bile duct. The common bile duct then releases them into the duodenum where they are activated to break down carbohydrates, fats, and proteins so that these substances may be more readily absorbed by the small intestine.

The digestive enzymes in the bicarbonate-rich fluid include trypsin, chymotrypsin, aminopeptidase, elastase, amylase, lipase phospholipases, and nucleases. This bicarbonate-rich fluid that the exocrine gland releases also neutralizes stomach acid in the duodenum.

HOW IS THE BLOOD GLUCOSE LEVEL REGULATED?

Due to the fact that glucose is the body's primary source of energy, its levels in the blood are tightly regulated. This blood glucose level is, as we know, regulated by insulin (which lowers it when it is too high), and glucagon, a peptide hormone made by the pancreas (which elevates the level of blood glucose when it is too low). Blood glucose levels increase following a meal, which signals the pancreas to release insulin into the bloodstream.

This signal involves the following steps: Glucose is transported from the blood to the beta-cells of the pancreas through a glucose transporter protein-2 (GLUT-2). Increased glucose levels in the beta-cells enhance production of ATP (adenosine triphosphate), resulting in an increase in the ATP/ADP (adeosine triphosphate/adenosine diphosphate) ratio. This leads to a closing of potassium+ channels (K+ channels), which causes depolarization of the cell membrane, which opens calcium channels. Opening of these calcium channels allows calcium to enter the beta-cells. Increased calcium levels in the beta-cells causes the release of insulin into the blood serum.

A diagramatic representation of this is presented in the box on page 6.

Elevated blood glucose level→→GLUT-2→→
Beta-cells→→Increases ATP→→Increases ratio of
ATP/ADP→→Closes potassium channels→→Depolarizes
beta-cells→→Opens calcium channels→→Calcium accumulates
in beta-cells→→Insulin secreted into the bloodstream.

GLUCOSE TRANSPORTER PROTEINS (GLUT)

In the same way that it is important to understand how insulin is produced and released into the bloodstream, it is also important to understand how glucose is transported from the blood into the cells. This job is done by glucose transporter proteins (GLUT), referenced above. There are four major types of glucose transporter proteins, GLUT-1, GLUT-2, GLUT-3, and GLUT-4.

1. **GLUT-1:** This type of GLUT is present in all human tissue, especially in red blood cells and blood vessels of the brain, and in fetal tissue. It has strong affinity for glucose, which assures a sufficient supply of glucose to the brain and red blood cells. GLUT-1 can transport galactose but not fructose.

2. **GLUT-2:** This type of GLUT is also present in all tissue; however, the pancreas, liver, kidneys, and small intestine contain the highest levels of GLUT-2. It is most active when blood glucose levels increase. It can transport galactose and fructose.

3. **GLUT-3:** This type of GLUT is primarily located in the brain, placenta, and testes and is the primary carrier of glucose for the nerve cells. Like GLUT-1, it can transport galactose but not fructose.

4. **GLUT-4:** This type of GLUT is also present in all cells, but it is present in abundance in heart muscle, skeletal muscle, adipocytes (fat cells), and the liver. Unlike other types of GLUT, GLUT-4 can transport only glucose. Insulin acts through its receptors

located on the cell surface of the target tissues. For example, insulin binds with its receptors on muscle cells. The receptor-bound insulin, through its intracellular signalling pathway, causes translocation (migration) of GLUT-4 from the Golgi apparatus to the cell membrane. Here it facilitates the uptake of glucose into the cells. In fat cells and muscle cells, if glucose is not needed for energy production, it is stored in the form of glycogen.

The binding of insulin to insulin receptors on liver cells also causes an increased synthesis of glycogen and inhibits glucose production by these cells. When circulating glucose decreases to a significant level, it triggers the release of glucagon from the alpha-cells of the pancreas. Glucagon then stimulates liver cells to produce more glucose, either by the breakdown of glycogen or by the production of new glucose from amino acids (National Diabetes Information Clearinghouse 2012).

THE GENESIS OF DIFFERENT TYPES OF DIABETES

As we have established, there are three main types of diabetes. We will elaborate on each of these next, to be followed by a discussion of the diabetes-related condition known as prediabetes, and a discussion of other types of diabetes as well.

Type 1 Diabetes and Its Possible Causes

Although type 1 diabetes is found most often in children and young adults, it can develop at any age. As mentioned previously, it is inherited from the parents as a genetic defect that causes a loss of insulin production by the pancreas. The pancreas does not produce sufficient insulin due to the progressive death of insulin-producing cells. Because the ensuing hyperglycemia requires daily injections of insulin in order that a normal blood glucose level is maintained, type 1 diabetes is also known as insulin-dependent diabetes. (Formerly type 1 diabetes was referred to as juvenile-onset diabetes.) It accounts for about 10 percent of all diabetes cases.

Although we don't know what causes the loss of insulin-producing beta-cells by the pancreas, three possibilities have been proposed. They include autoimmunity, genetic susceptibility, and environmental insult.

Autoimmunity

Although the symptoms of type 1 diabetes appear suddenly, it is thought that this form of the disease is caused by a chronic attack on beta-cells by the body's own immune cells over a period of many years. Clinical symptoms of type 1 diabetes, such as hyperglycemia, appear after more than 90 percent of the beta-cells have been destroyed. The involvement of immune-mediated damage to beta-cells is supported by the fact that immunosuppressive treatment produced beneficial effects in experimental animals and in children with the new onset of type 1 diabetes (Crawford and Cotran 1999).

The exact reasons for the development of autoimmunity are unknown. Increased oxidative stress damages DNA, RNA, proteins, and lipids. These damaged biological molecules are normally removed from the body. If they are not removed, they may act as an antigen (foreign agent) that evokes an immune response designed to remove them by producing target-cell-specific antibodies. For example, in response to damaged beta-cell-specific proteins that had not been removed, immune cells may produce antibodies that can further damage the beta-cells, eventually causing them to die.

Genetic Susceptibility

Type 1 diabetes is commonly found in people of northern European descent. Other ethnic groups such as African Americans, Native Americans, and Asian Americans have a much lower incidence of this form of diabetes. One of the susceptibile genes for type 1 diabetes is the human leukocyte antigen-D (HLA-D), also called the major histocompatibilty complex (MHC).

Environmental Insult

Epidemiologic (survey-type) studies suggest that certain viruses such as the coxsackie virus, mumps, measles, cytomagalovirus, rubella, and the Epstein-Barr virus (infectious mononucleosis) may be associated with type 1 diabetes. One of the ways that viruses may induce type 1 diabetes involves direct injury to beta-cells, which evokes autoimmune reactions that then kill beta-cells. Other possible environmental factors include a young child's ingestion of cow's milk prior to the age of four, and some drugs such as pentamidine—commonly used to treat parasitic infections—and the accidental or intentional ingestion of Vacor, a pharmacological agent used to exterminate rats.

It is unfortunate that, at present, there are no strategies to reduce the risk and development of type 1 diabetes in children. However, a laboratory study has shown that daily supplementation with an appropriate multiple antioxidant has prevented the genetic basis of some diseases such as cancer (Prasad 2011). (We will elaborate on this finding in chapter 8.) Therefore, it is possible that an appropriate micronutrient* preparation containing multiple dietary and endogenous antioxidants, taken regularly by a child older than three, may prevent or delay the onset of type 1 diabetes. It is also possible that this same strategy may work for a pregnant woman in order to prevent the onset of type 1 diabetes in her child.

Type 2 Diabetes and Its Possible Causes

Type 2 diabetes is called non-insulin-dependent diabetes, previously referred to as adult-onset diabetes. It generally occurs in older individuals but it is appearing at increasing rates among children and adolescents, especially among African Americans, Latinos, and Pacific Islanders. Considered an acquired disease, not an inherited one (as is

---

*Micronutrients include antioxidants, B vitamins, vitamin D, and certain minerals such as selenium and zinc.

type 1), it accounts for about 80 to 90 percent of all existing cases of diabetes.

When type 2 diabetes is diagnosed, the pancreas is usually producing adequate amounts of insulin; however, the tissues of the body cannot use it efficiently. This condition of insulin resistance causes hyperglycemia. (Over time, chronic hyperglycemia can gradually damage beta-cells of the pancreas by generating excessive amounts of free radicals that would reduce the production and/or release of insulin.)

Although the reasons for the development of insulin resistance are generally not well understood, in my opinon there are at least two potential contributing factors for it. As we have previously discussed, insulin binds with insulin receptors that are located on the surface of the cells. The receptor-bound insulin, through a series of steps, causes glucose tranporting proteins (GLUTs) to migrate from the Golgi apparatus to the cell membrane, where they facilitate the uptake of glucose inside the cells. If the insulin receptors are damaged by free radicals, GLUTs theoretically are not able to relocate from the Golgi apparatus to the cell membrane, which would then prevent or reduce the uptake of glucose by the cells.

Glucose transporter proteins can also be damaged by free radicals while present in the cell membrane, which would interfere with the uptake of glucose by the cells. Thus, damage to the insulin receptors and/or GLUTs may account for the development of insulin resistance, which eventually can lead to type 2 diabetes.

Major risk factors for type 2 diabetes include obesity and a lack of physical activity, genetic susceptibility, insulin resistance, excess production of glucose by the liver, and age and ethnicity.

Obesity and a Lack of Physical Activity

Obesity and physical inactivity are some of the greatest contributing factors to the development of type 2 diabetes. The excessive consumption of carbohydrates and fats, together with a lack of physical activity, can cause obesity—and generally if caloric intake is higher than caloric loss, obesity may result after a few years. Abdominal fat deposits are considered one of the predictors of the development of type 2 diabetes. Excess abdominal fat (belly fat) also produces excessive amounts of pro-inflammatory cytokines (interleukin-6 and tumor necosis factor-alpha), free fatty acids (increase blood levels of lipids), and interferes with the normal function of hormones leptin (normally dampens appetite) and adiponectin (normally influences response of cell to insulin). Additionally, an excessive intake of total calories and fat is known to generate excessive amounts of free radicals in the body. These risk factors *can* be changed in order to reduce the risk of developing type 2 diabetes.

Genetic Susceptibility

Type 2 diabetes is the result of an interaction between genes and the environment. About forty genes appear to be associated with type 2 diabetes. Most of these genes affect insulin secretion from the pancreas; however, a few of them are associated with decreased insulin sensitivity and obesity (Kahn et al. 2012).

Insulin is stored within the secretory vesicles or granules inside the beta-cells in the pancreas. Exocytosis is a process by which the beta-cells release this stored insulin from the granules. Defects in the exocytosis of beta-cells can reduce the release of insulin into the bloodstream. Among twenty-three exocytotic genes, the levels of STX1A protein (syntaxin-1A protein) encoded by the gene STX1A, SYT4 protein (synaptotagmin-4 protein) encoded by the SYT4 gene, and SYT 11 were reduced in patients with type 2 diabetes (Andersson et al. 2012).

It has been reported that the expression of four genes involved in oxidative phosphorylation were reduced in patients with type 2 diabetes. These genes were NDUFA-5 (NADH-ubiquinone oxidoreductase 1 alpha-subunit-5), NADUFA-10, COX-11 (cytochrome oxidase-c-subunit-11), and ATP6V1H. An elevated expression of the calpain gene is correlated with an increased release of insulin from beta-cells in non-diabetic individuals, but this capacity of calpain was lost in patients with type 2 diabetes (Ling et al. 2009).

Transcriptional factor 7-like 2 (TCF7L2), a key element of the Wnt (integration gene in wingless fruit flies), regulates the secretion of insulin from the beta-cells of the pancreas. This gene increases the risk of type 2 diabetes in all ethnic groups. The presence of this gene in an individual increases the risk of this form of diabetes by 50 percent (Cauchi and Froguel 2008).

These selected studies suggest that changes in gene activity play an important role in the development of type 2 diabetes. These genetic risk factors *cannot* be changed by most preventive strategies.

Insulin Resistance

Chronic insulin resistance can lead to type 2 diabetes. Insulin resistance may develop due to the following reasons:

1. Defects in insulin receptors caused by free radicals or a genetic defect
2. Defects in glucose tranporter proteins caused by free radicals or a genetic defect

These defects can be used as targets for prevention strategies designed to mitigate the development of this form of diabetes.

Excess Production of Glucose by the Liver

In some patients with type 2 diabetes, excessive production of glucose by the liver is a causative factor. Normally, when blood glucose and insulin levels are low, the pancreas releases glucagon, which stimulates the liver to produce glucose and release it into the bloodstream. When levels of blood glucose and insulin are high, the levels of glucagon decrease. However, in some individuals, glucagon levels remain consistently high, which signals the liver to produce more glucose, even though it is not needed. This causes blood glucose levels to rise, leading to hyperglycemia.

Age and Ethnicity

Older individuals are at a greater risk for developing type 2 diabetes. As stated earlier, African Americans, Latinos, and Pacific Islanders are at a higher risk of developing type 2 diabetes compared to Caucasians.

These risk factors *cannot* be changed by the individuals.

Gestational Diabetes

As discussed previously, although gestational diabetes presents in pregnant women, it typically resolves after the baby is born. However, with these women there remains a 35 to 60 percent chance that they will develop diabetes in the next ten to twenty years. Using new diagnostic tools and criteria, it has been determined that 18 percent of pregnancies are affected by gestational diabetes and immediately following pregnancy, 5 to 10 percent of women with gestational diabetes are found to have diabetes, typically type 2 (National Diabetes Information Clearinghouse 2012).

Related Conditions and Other Types of Diabetes

In addition to the three major types of diabetes, the condition known as prediabetes exists, which is just as its name implies.

There are other types of diabetes as well. They include defects in the immune system and mutations (changes) in one or more genes of the beta-cells. Diabetes can also be induced by injury to the pancreas (pancreatitis), infection, cancer of the pancreas, cystic fibrosis, and/or hemochromatosis (a disease of iron overload in the body). It can also be caused by the excessive presence of certain hormones such as growth hormone in acromegalies, cortisol in Cushing's syndrome, glucagon in glucagonoma, and epinephrine in pheochromocytoma. We will examine the condition known as prediabetes, as well as some of the above-referenced forms of diabetes, more closely now.

Prediabetes

Persons with prediabetes exhibit higher than normal blood sugar levels but these levels are not high enough to categorize them as diabetic. A prediabetic condition is also referred to as impaired fasting glucose (IFG). The blood glucose level after overnight fasting is 100–125 milligrams/dL in individuals with prediabetes. These individuals are likely to develop type 2 diabetes within ten years. They are also at higher risk for developing heart disease and stroke.

The incidence of prediabetes is increasing in the United States. The U.S. Department of Health and Human Services estimated that in 2007, at least 57 million American adults age twenty or older had prediabetes. In 2010, the total number of people with prediabetes had risen to 79 million, an increase of approximately 38.5 percent.

Latent Autoimmune Diabetes in Adults

In latent autoimmune diabetes in adults (LADA), individuals may exhibit signs of both type 1 and type 2 diabetes. LADA is generally seen in individuals who are older than thirty. Researchers have estimated that about 10 percent of individuals diagnosed with type 2 diabetes actually have LADA. Patients with LADA have antibodies targeting the beta-cells of the pancreas, thus resembling type 1 diabetes. Most patients with LADA are producing their own insulin at the time of their diagnosis.

Genetic Defects in Beta-cells

Genetic defects in beta-cells cause a monogenic form of diabetes that results from a defect in a single gene. There are two major forms of monogenic diabetes: maturity-onset diabetes of the young (MODY), and neonatal diabetes mellitus (NDM). This gene defect is passed on from one generation to another. MODY generally occurs during early childhood and is associated with a number of different gene defects, all of which reduce the ability of beta-cells to produce insulin. NDM generally occurs within six months of the birth of the baby. In this form of diabetes, the beta-cells do not produce sufficient amounts of insulin. It can be mistaken for type 1 diabetes.

Genetic Defects in Insulin Action

Insulin acts through the insulin receptors that are located on the surface of the cells. Genetic defects in insulin receptors may interfere with the action of insulin, thereby decreasing blood levels of glucose.

COMPLICATIONS RELATED TO DIABETES

Complications related to diabetes include increased risk of heart disease and stroke, hypertension, eye problems, kidney disease, damage to the nervous system (impaired sensations or pain in the hands or feet, the slowed digestion of food, erectile dysfunction), gum disease, hearing loss, birth defects, amputation of the lower limbs, dental disease, complications of pregnancy, and biochemical imbalances that can cause acute life-threatening events, including coma. We will discuss some of these complications next.

Heart Disease and Stroke

In 2004, heart disease was found in 68 percent of diabetes-related death certificates among those individuals age sixty-five or older. Stroke was noted in 16 percent of the same group. Death rates from heart disease and stroke are two to four times higher in patients with diabetes than those without diabetes.

Hypertension

From 2006 to 2008, 67 percent of diabetic patients age twenty or older had hypertension. Their levels of blood pressure were equal to or greater than 140/90 millimeters of mercury (mmHg). (Normal blood pressure value is 120/80.)

Eye Problems

Diabetes is the leading cause of blindness among people between the ages of twenty and seventy-four. From 2005 to 2008, 28.5 percent of patients with diabetes (4.2 million) had retinopathy (damage to the eyes) and among them 4.4 percent (655,000) had severe retinopathy, which can lead to vision loss.

Kidney Disease

Diabetes is also the leading cause of kidney failure, accounting for approximately 44 percent of all new cases of it in 2005. End-stage kidney disease affected 48,374 persons with diabetes in 2008; a total of 202,290 individuals were living on chronic dialysis or with kidney transplants.

Damage to the Nervous System

It has been estimated that approximately 60–70 percent of diabetic patients have mild to severe forms of neuropathy. About 30 percent of patients with diabetes age forty or older have impaired sensations in the feet. Severe forms of nerve damage among patients with diabetes may lead to a deleterious condition requiring the amputation of a lower limb. It has been estimated that more than 60 percent of non-traumatic lower-limb amputations occur in patients with diabetes. Non-traumatic amputations performed in diabetic patients in 2006 numbered 65,700.

Gum Disease

The risk of developing periodontis in patients with diabetes is two times greater than for those who do not have diabetes. It has been estimated that about one-third of patients with diabetes have severe gum disease.

Hearing Loss

Data obtained from the National Health Nutrition Examination Survey (1999–2004) involving 5,140 participants showed that approximately 21 percent of individuals with diabetes had hearing loss, whereas only 9 percent of individuals without diabetes had hearing loss (Bainbridge et al. 2008). This increase in hearing loss among patients with diabetes was independent of other risk factors such as intense noise and ototoxic medications (damage to ear cells causing hearing loss). This finding was confirmed by another survey-type study in which 165 patients with diabetes and 137 individuals without diabetes were randomly selected to determine the association between diabetes and hearing loss. The results showed that diabetes *was* associated with hearing loss. Furthermore, it was more pronounced in individuals less than fifty years of age (Austin et al. 2009).

Birth Defects

Researchers have shown that poorly controlled diabetes before pregnancy or during the first trimester is associated with birth defects in about 5–10 percent of pregnancies, and spontaneous abortions in about 15–20 percent of pregnancies. Poorly controlled diabetes during the second and third trimesters can lead to the birth of excessively large babies, which can increase the health risks for both mother and baby.

METABOLIC SYNDROME, A PRECURSOR TO TYPE 2 DIABETES

Increased oxidative stress and chronic inflammation are among the major biochemical factors that may play an important role in the initiation and progression of type 1 and type 2 diabetes. Oxidative stress and chronic inflammation also play a significant role in the development of metabolic syndrome, also known as insulin resistance syndrome. Metabolic syndrome is a cluster of criteria that helps doctors to identify who may be at risk for the development of serious health problems. Because it may be an important marker for the development of type 2 diabetes, we will elaborate on it here before turning our attention more fully to oxidative stress and chronic inflammation in the next chapter of this book.

Markers of Metabolic Syndrome

The manifestation of three or more of the criteria (risk factors) for metabolic syndrome cited below makes one vulnerable to health problems such as diabetes, stroke, and heart disease.

The National Cholesterol Education Program's Adult Treatment Panel III (NCEP/ATP III) has proposed the following guidelines to identify people with metabolic syndrome:

Abdominal obesity (waist circumference) in men	Greater than 102 centimeters (40 inches)
Abdominal obesity (waist circumference) in women	Greater than 88 centimeters (35 inches)
Triglycerides	150 mg/dL or more
HDL cholesterol in men	less than 40 mg/dL
HDL cholesterol in women	less than 50 mg/dL
Blood pressure	135/85 mm Hg or more
Fasting glucose	100 mg/dL or more

Incidence of Metabolic Syndrome

The incidence of metabolic syndrome varies depending upon age, gender, and ethnicity. It is increasing in the United States, where it is found in approximately 34 percent of the population age twenty or older (Ervin 2009). About 53 percent of individuals with metabolic syndrome have abdominal obesity, 40 percent have high blood pressure, 35 percent have high triglycerides, and 25 percent have low HDL cholesterol.

The incidence of metabolic syndrome is threefold higher among men and women age forty to forty-nine, it is fourfold higher among men who are sixty and older, and it is sixfold higher among women age sixty and older compared to younger individuals between the ages of twenty and thirty-nine.

The incidence of metabolic syndrome among non-Latino African-American males was 50 percent of that observed among non-Latino Caucasian men. Among non-Latinos, African Americans, and Latino-American women, it was one and a half times higher compared to non-Latino Caucasian women.

The incidence of metabolic syndrome was sixfold higher among overweight men, whereas it was thirty-two times higher among obese men compared to men of normal weight. The incidence of metabolic syndrome was five times higher among overweight women whereas it was seventeen times higher among obese women compared to women of normal weight.

Risk Factors for Metabolic Syndrome

The most important risk factors for metabolic syndrome include abdominal obesity and insulin resistance. Other risk factors include age, race, gender, and physical inactivity. Certain risk factors such as obesity, insulin resistance, and physical inactivity can be changed to reduce the risk of metabolic syndrome. Others such as age, race, and gender cannot.

As noted earlier, metabolic syndrome may be a possible precursor to the development of type 2 diabetes, for as we know, increased oxidative stress occurs in individuals manifesting some of its defined characteristics. Increased levels of insulin and impaired glycemic control were associated with higher levels of oxidized low-density lipids (LDL) in patients with metabolic syndrome (Holvoet 2008).

In a clinical study involving forty-three individuals with metabolic syndrome without type 2 diabetes and thirty-three healthy individuals without metabolic syndrome, the blood levels of markers of oxidative stress were determined. The results showed that the release of free radicals (superoxide anion) from monocytes was enhanced in individuals with metabolic syndrome compared to individuals without metabolic syndrome. The expression of NADPH oxidase on the cell membrane was also increased in subjects with metabolic syndrome compared to those without it.

Furthermore, the levels of nuclear factor erythroid 2-related factor (involved in cellular antioxidant defense) decreased in monocytes obtained from the individuals with metabolic syndrome compared to those without it. The plasma levels of nitrotyrosine (tyrosine, an amino acid damaged by free radicals derived from nitrogen) and oxidized LDL cholesterol (markers of increased oxidative stress) were elevated in patients with metabolic syndrome compared to those without it (Jialal et al. 2012).

Survey of data from the National Health and Nutrition Survey (NHANES) 2001–2006 revealed that the incidence of metabolic syndrome among adolescents between the ages of twelve and nineteen was 7 percent for boys and 3 percent for girls. Lower levels of carotenoids were associated with insulin resistance and higher levels of C-reactive protein in patients with metabolic syndrome. Vitamin C level was also lower in patients with metabolic syndrome than those without metabolic syndrome. Vitamin E levels in plasma were found to have no association with metabolic syndrome (Beydoun et al. 2012).

Adiponectin is a protein hormone secreted by fat cells. It helps regulate plasma levels of glucose and breaks down fatty acids. The level of adiponectin decreased and the level of MDA increased in patients with metabolic syndrome (Sankhla et al. 2012). A series of recent studies also supports the role of increased oxidative stress in the development and progression of metabolic syndrome (Aroor et al. 2012; Pietropaoli et al. 2012; Venturini et al. 2012).

CONCLUDING REMARKS

Diabetes is a chronic disease wherein elevated plasma levels of glucose exist in the body due to a lack of insulin production by the pancreas, and/or because the body has become resistant to insulin. The incidence and cost of this disease continue to increase throughout the world, necessitating an effective treatment strategy to mitigage its onset and development.

Type 1 diabetes (insulin-dependent diabetes) makes up approximately 10 percent of all diabetic cases. It is caused by the pancreas's inability to generate the beta-cells that produce insulin. Although it can develop at any age, type 1 diabetes is most often found in children and young adults.

Type 2 diabetes (non-insulin-dependent diabetes, previously referred to as adult-onset diabetes) makes up roughly 80–90 percent of all cases of diabetes. Although it generally manifests in older persons, its prevalence among children and teenagers is increasing.

Gestational diabetes occurs only in pregnant women who develop it late in pregnancy. Although it often resolves following the birth of the child, the pregnant woman is at greater risk for developing type 2 diabetes.

A condition related to diabetes, called prediabetes, is, like type 2 diabetes, also on the rise. Metabolic syndrome is another associated condition. It is characterized by high blood pressure, high blood sugar levels, excessive fat around the waist, and high cholesterol levels.

Heart disease, hypertension, eye problems, kidney failure, and damage to the nervous system are all diabetes-related complications.

Factors which predispose one for type 1 diabetes include autoimmunity, genetic susceptibility, and environmental insults. Risk factors for type 2 diabetes include obesity and physical inactivity, genetic susceptibility, insulin resistance, excess production of glucose by the liver, age and ethnicity, and defects in insulin receptors and glucose transporter proteins.

We will explore the additional contributing factors of oxidative stress and chronic inflammation in the next chapter, before elaborating on our envisioned prevention and improved management protocols in the following pages of this book.

2 Oxidative Stress and Inflammation

Compounding Factors of Diabetes

The external and internal causes contributing to the development and onset of diabetes are manifold, and typically generate excessive amounts of free radicals in the body. In turn, these free radicals contribute to an increase in oxidative stress and chronic inflammation, which are largely responsible for the development of diabetes and the diabetes-related complications of retinopathy (damage to the eyes), neuropathy (damage to the nerves, such as a numbness of the extremities), and nephropathy (damage to the kidneys).

In the context of our broader discussion about diabetes, it is essential to become familiar with the processes of oxidative stress and inflammation—both chronic and acute—and the key role that free radicals play in both. Let's take a look at free radicals first.

FREE RADICALS

Free radicals are atoms, molecules, or ions with unpaired electrons, and can be derived either from oxygen or nitrogen. In 1900, the first organic free radical, triphenylmethyl radical, was identified by Moses Gomberg of the University of Michigan. Free radicals are symbolized by a dot "•". When the levels of free radicals in the body exceed the antioxidant capacity of the body to neutralize them, oxidative stress occurs. Increased oxidative stress causes damage to cells and tissues, including cellular structures such as DNA (deoxyribonucleic acid), RNA (ribonucleic acid), proteins, fat, and membranes.

Our body produces different types of free radicals, the half-lives* of which can vary from 10^{-9} seconds (most are quickly destroyed after causing damage), to days, as you can ascertain from the information in the box below.

The Half-Lives of Some Free Radicals

Hydroxyl = 10^{-9} seconds

Superoxide anion = 10^{-5} seconds

Nitric oxide = about 1 second

Lipid peroxyl = 7 seconds

Hydrogen peroxide = minutes

Semiquinone = days

The sources and methods of the production of free radicals are varied.

OXIDATIVE STRESS: REDUCTION AND OXIDATION PROCESSES IN THE BODY

To understand the role of free radicals and antioxidants it is important to grasp the relationship between the processes of reduction and oxidation, which are constantly taking place in the human body.

Reduction

Reduction is a process in which an atom or molecule loses oxygen, gains hydrogen, or gains an electron. For example, carbon dioxide loses

---

*A half-life is the time needed to remove a substance from the blood, divided by two.

oxygen and becomes carbon monoxide, carbon gains hydrogen and becomes methane, and oxygen gains an electron and becomes a superoxide anion. Thus, a *reducing agent* is an atom or molecule that changes another chemical by removing oxygen from it or by adding an electron or hydrogen to it. All antioxidants can be considered reducing agents. An elevated level of antioxidants in the body inclines the body to favor the reduction process over the oxidation process, thereby keeping it healthy.

Oxidation

Oxidation is a process by which an atom or molecule either gains oxygen, loses hydrogen, or loses an electron. For example, carbon gains oxygen during oxidation and becomes carbon dioxide. A superoxide radical loses an electron during the oxidation process and becomes oxygen. Thus, an *oxidizing agent* is an atom or molecule that changes another chemical by adding oxygen to it or by removing an electron or hydrogen from it. Examples of oxidizing agents include free radicals, X-rays, and ozone. Oxidizing agents *that are formed in the body,* in addition to free radicals, include peroxynitrite, hydrogen peroxide, and lipid peroxide, all of which are very damaging to the cells of the body. It should also be noted that an oxidized antioxidant (one that has been damaged by free radicals) acts as a pro-oxidant (like a free radical) rather than as an antioxidant.

Oxidative Stress and Nitrosylative Stress

As we know, oxidative stress refers to a condition in which the increased production of free radicals derived from oxygen occurs. Nitrosylative stress, on the other hand, refers to a condition in which the increased production of free radicals derived from *nitrogen* occurs. Both increased oxidative stress and nitrosylative stress increase the risk of chronic diseases.

Processes Involving Oxygen and Nitrogen in the Production of Free Radicals

The formative process of some *reactive oxygen species (ROS: free radicals derived from oxygen)* is described below.

When molecular oxygen (O_2) acquires an electron, the superoxide anion ($O_2^{\bullet-}$) is formed:

$$O_2 + e^- = O_2^{\bullet-}$$

Superoxide dismutase (SOD) and H^+ can react with $O_2^{\bullet-}$ to form hydrogen peroxide (H_2O_2):

$$2O_2^{\bullet-} + 2H^+ \text{ plus SOD} \rightarrow H_2O_2 + O_2$$
$$O_2^{\bullet-} + H^+ \rightarrow HO_2^{\bullet} \text{ (hydroxyl radical)}$$
$$2HO_2^{\bullet} \rightarrow H_2O_2 + O_2$$

Ferric and ferrous forms of iron can react with superoxide anion and hydrogen peroxide to produce molecular oxygen (O_2) and hydroxyl radicals ($OH^{\bullet}$), respectively:

$$Fe^{3+} + O_2^{\bullet-} \rightarrow Fe^{2+} + O_2$$
$$Fe^{2+} + H_2O_2 \rightarrow Fe^{3+} + OH^{\bullet} + OH^- \text{ (Fenton reaction)}$$

Hydroxyl radicals can also be formed from superoxide anion by the Haber-Weiss reaction:

$$O_2^{\bullet-} + H_2O_2 \rightarrow O_2 + OH^- + OH^{\bullet}$$

Both the Fenton and Haber-Weiss reactions require a transition metal such as copper or iron. Among ROS, $OH^{\bullet}$ is the most damaging free radical and is very short-lived.

Hydroxyl radicals are very reactive with a variety of organic compounds, leading to the production of more radical compounds:

$$RH \text{ (organic compound)} + OH^\bullet \rightarrow R^\bullet \text{ (organic radical)} + H_2O$$

$$R^\bullet + O_2 \rightarrow RO_2^\bullet \text{ (peroxyl radical)}$$

For example, the DNA radical can be generated by reaction with a hydroxyl radical, and this can lead to a break in the DNA strand.

Catalase detoxifies hydrogen peroxide to form water and molecular oxygen:

$$H_2O_2 + catalase \rightarrow H_2O \text{ and } O_2$$

Reactive *nitrogen species (RNS: free radicals derived from nitrogen)* are represented by nitric oxide (NO$^\bullet$). NO is synthesized by the enzyme nitric oxide synthase from L-arginine. NO$^\bullet$ can combine with superoxide anion to form peroxynitrite, a powerful oxidant:

$$NO^\bullet + O_2^{\bullet-} \rightarrow ONOO^- \text{ (peroxynitrite)}$$

When protonated (likely at physiological pH), peroxynitrite spontaneously decomposes to reactive nitric dioxide and hydroxyl radicals:

$$ONOO^- + H^+ \rightarrow {}^\bullet NO_2 + OH^\bullet$$

Superoxide dismutase (SOD) can also enhance the peroxynitrite-mediated nitration of tyrosine residues on critical proteins, presumably via species similar to the nitronium cation (NO$_2^+$):

$$ONOO^- \text{ plus SOD} \rightarrow NO_2^+ \rightarrow \text{Nitration of tyrosine}$$

Other Processes That Produce Free Radicals

Mitochondria are elongated membranous structures in the cells. As they generate energy with the help of oxygen, mitochondria produce certain types of free radicals (superoxide anions and hydroxyl radicals) as by-products. During this process, about 2 percent of unused oxygen leaks out of the mitochondria and makes about 20 billion molecules of superoxide anions and hydrogen peroxide per cell per day.

Free radicals are also generated in the course of a bacterial or viral infection wherein phagocytic cells (a kind of white blood cell) engulf invading microorganisms and generate high levels of nitric oxide, superoxide anions, and hydrogen peroxide in order to kill infectious organisms. Excessive production of free radicals by phagocytes can also damage normal cells.

As well, in the course of the metabolism of fatty acids and other molecules in the body, free radicals are produced. Certain habits such as tobacco smoking, and the presence of trace minerals of free iron, copper, and manganese in the body can also increase the rate of production of free radicals. Free radicals are also formed by the consequences of obesity, exposure to ionizing radiation such as X-rays, the aging process, and the excessive use of oxygen, such as during aerobic exercise.

As we can see, the human body is constantly exposed to varying levels of damaging free radicals that are derived from many different sources. Fortunately, we are endowed with an antioxidant defense system that protects the body against this damage. However, this defense system may not be effective if the production of free radicals is so excessive as to overwhelm the system and impact its ability to function successfully in protecting the body from disease and decay.

INCREASED OXIDATIVE STRESS IN DIABETES

Increased oxidative stress is a major biochemical factor that may play an important role in the initiation and progression of both type 1 and type 2 diabetes, as well as in metabolic syndrome, and indeed, extensive animal and human studies bear this out. Markers of oxidative stress that can be detected in the blood are elevated in patients with diabetes and metabolic syndrome. An excessive intake of glucose increases the activity of the NADPH oxidase enzyme, which converts molecular oxygen to free radicals (superoxide anion). Hyperglycemia also damages mitochondria, and damaged mitochondria produce increased amounts of free radicals.

Some selected studies on changes in the markers of oxidative stress in type 1 and type 2 diabetes are briefly described here.

Evidence of Increased Oxidative Stress in Type 1 Diabetes

The results of several human and animal studies suggest that markers of oxidative stress are elevated in children with type 1 diabetes (Martin-Gallan et al. 2003).

It has been shown that hyperglycemia-induced oxidative stress may play an important role in the progression of type 1 diabetes (Cinkilic et al. 2009).

In another clinical study, the levels of markers of protein glycation and oxidative stress in blood and serum were determined in the following groups:

1. Eighty-one patients with type 1 diabetes, involving sixty-one patients with poor long-term glycemic (glucose) control and twenty patients with good long-term glycemic control
2. Thirty-one healthy children (control group)

The results showed that the levels of glycation end-products and advanced oxidation protein products in diabetic patients were higher compared to the control group. The highest levels were found in patients with poor glycemic control (Kostolanska et al. 2009).

These studies suggest that increased oxidative stress plays an important role in the progression of type 1 diabetes.

Patients with type 1 diabetes rely on insulin injections for maintaining normal glucose levels in the body. Despite this treatment, most eventually develop insulin resistance and other symptoms of type 2 diabetes. The exact mechanisms of this are unknown; however, increased oxidative stress may be one of the factors in the development of insulin resistance.

This is supported by the fact that prolonged treatment of cultured mouse hepatocytes (liver cells) with insulin increased oxidative stress.

In addition, insulin resistance was associated with impaired mitochondrial function. It was demonstrated that overexpression of an antioxidant enzyme mitochondrial MnSOD (manganese-dependent superoxide dismutase) prevented insulin-induced insulin resistance (Liu et al. 2009).

In order to further demonstrate the role of oxidative stress in the development and progression of type 1 diabetes, a clinical study evaluated the levels of markers of oxidative stress and antioxidant systems in the following groups:

1. Twenty children with type 1 diabetes
2. Twenty-two obese children with no diabetes
3. Sixteen age-sex-matched control children with no diabetes

The results of the above study revealed the following:

1. The levels of markers of oxidative stress such as lipoperoxides (oxidized lipid), malondialdehyde (MDA), and protein oxidation were significantly higher in both patients with diabetes and obese children, compared to the control group.
2. The level of MDA was highest in children with diabetes.
3. The serum levels of alpha-tocopherol, beta-carotene, glutathione, and the activity of the antioxidant enzyme glutathione peroxidase in patients with diabetes were lower compared to obese children with no diabetes.

From these results, it was concluded that oxidative stress is elevated in both children with type 1 diabetes and obesity (Codoner-Franch et al. 2010).

However, it is not certain whether increased oxidative stress precedes or merely reflects the consequences of this disease. In order to clarify this issue, a clinical study was performed to evaluate the levels of markers of oxidative stress in the following groups:

1. Thirty patients with type 1 diabetes, involving ten without diabetic complications, ten with retinopathy (eye damage), and ten with nephropathy (kidney damage)
2. Thirty-six non-diabetic siblings
3. Thirty-seven non-diabetic parents of type 1 diabetic patients
4. Three healthy subjects without a familial history of diabetes (control group)

The following results were obtained:

1. The levels of MDA (a marker of oxidative stress) in plasma and red blood cells (RBCs) were elevated in diabetic patients and their relatives (non-diabetic siblings and non-diabetic parents of type 1 diabetes patients) compared to the control group.
2. The levels of the antioxidant glutathione in red blood cells were lower in diabetic patients and their relatives compared to the control group, which did not have a family history of diabetes.

The results showed that increased oxidative stress occurs in non-diabetic relatives of diabetic patients, therefore, increased oxidative stress may precede the development of type 1 diabetes (Matteucci and Giampietro 2000). This study is important because it suggests that increased oxidative stress may be one of the important factors in the development of type 1 diabetes.

In a clinical study involving fifty-nine patients with type 1 diabetes, it was observed that lower plasma vitamin C levels were associated with blood-vessel dysfunction (Odermarsky et al. 2009). Lower plasma levels of vitamin C may cause increased oxidative stress in these patients and may be responsible for harmful changes in blood vessels.

Streptozotocin treatment induces diabetes in rats. In these diabetic rats, the activity of the enzyme NADPH oxidase-4 and the level of gene NOX-4 that codes for this enzyme were elevated. The levels of free radicals were also elevated. The markers of cardiomyopathy (damage to the heart muscle) such as fibronectin, collagen, alpha-smooth muscle actin, and the beta-myosin heavy chain were also increased. Furthermore, treatment of cardiac myocytes (heart muscle cells) in a culture with high-dose glucose increased the activity of NADPH oxidase, the level of NOX-4 gene, and the above markers of heart-muscle cell damage. From this study, it was concluded that NOX-4 gene activity is an important source of free radicals, and that these specific free radicals contribute to the development of cardiomyopathy (a form of heart disease) at early stages of type 1 diabetes (Maalouf et al. 2012).

In type 1 diabetes patients, immunoglobulin G (IgG) is damaged by free radicals. The damaged IgG is called oxidized IgG. Circulating autoantibodies bind more readily with oxidized IgG than with normal IgG. In a clinical study, the binding of autoantibodies with oxidized IgG was compared between two groups: diabetic smokers (twenty-eight patients) and diabetic non-smokers (twenty-six patients). The results showed that the binding of antibodies with oxidized IgG was much higher in diabetic smokers than that in diabetic non-smokers. Normal human serum showed negligible binding of autoantibodies with either normal or oxidized IgG. Diabetic smokers showed higher levels of protein carbonyl (a protein marker of oxidative damage) than diabetic non-smokers. From these results, it was concluded that the oxidation of plasma proteins, especially IgG, may increase the progression of disease in type 1 diabetic smokers (Rasheed et al. 2011).

It has been suggested that the lower bone density found in children with type 1 diabetes is due to poor glucose control and increased oxidative stress (Heilman et al. 2009).

In a clinical study involving thirty-eight women with type 1 diabetes and twenty-five matched non-diabetic females, it was observed that initial increases in the markers of oxidative stress were associated with a decrease in the level of plasma uric acid (Pitocco et al. 2008).

Another clinical study involving twenty-seven young patients with type 1 diabetes and thirty-eight young non-diabetic patients found that increased oxidative stress and increased risk of vascular complications (damage to the blood vessels) were present in the early stages of type 1 diabetes (Hata et al. 2006).

The studies discussed above demonstrate that increased oxidative stress plays an important role in the development and progression of type 1 diabetes. Increased oxidative stress also contributes to the development of diabetes-related complications.

Evidence of Increased Oxidative Stress in Type 2 Diabetes

To demonstrate the role of oxidative damage in type 2 diabetes, a clinical study was performed to measure the levels of markers of oxidative stress and DNA damage in the following groups of patients:

1. Ninety-two subjects with normal glucose tolerance (NGT)
2. Seventy-eight patients with impaired glucose tolerance (IGT)
3. One hundred thirteen patients with newly diagnosed diabetes

The results of the study above showed that patients with impaired glucose tolerance displayed reduced activity of the antioxidant enzyme superoxide dismutase (SOD) in erythrocytes compared to patients with normal glucose tolerance. The patients with newly diagnosed diabetes had higher levels of plasma MDA (a marker of oxidative damage), and lower levels of total antioxidative capacity (TAC) and erythrocyte SOD activity than the patients with normal glucose tolerance. Damage to DNA was mild in patients with impaired glucose tolerance, but the level of DNA damage increased in patients with diabetes (Song et al. 2007).

Several studies have confirmed the fact that diabetes-related complications such as microalbuminuria (excess secretion of the protein albumin in the urine, a sign of kidney damage), periodontal disease (gum disease), nephropathy (damage to the kidneys), retinopathy (damage to the eyes), and cardiovascular disease (heart disease) are due to increased oxidative stress induced by hyperglycemia (El-Mesallamy et al. 2010; Mellor et al. 2010; Morales-Indiano et al. 2009).

The enzyme NAD (P) H oxidase is a major source of reactive oxygen species, and it is coded by the NOX-4 gene. This enzyme is localized in the mitochondria of many cells, including in the kidneys of diabetic rats. In another study, the expression of mitochondrial NOX-4 was elevated in the kidney cortex of diabetic rats, suggesting that NOX-4 is a major source of reactive oxygen species (ROS) in the kidneys during the early stages of diabetes (Block et al. 2009; Gorin et al. 2005). Thus, NOX-4-derived ROS contributes to renal hypertrophy (increase in the size of kidney cells) (Gorin et al. 2005).

In diabetic mice, it was shown that the development of type 2 diabetes–related nephropathy (kidney disease) was due to the production of excessive amounts of free radicals by NADPH oxidase (Sedeek et al. 2010).

It has been reported that in type 2 diabetic mice, exercise capacity and mitochondrial function in skeletal muscle were impaired due to increased oxidative stress (Yokota et al. 2009).

To evaluate the role increased oxidative stress plays in the development of insulin resistance in obese children, a clinical study was performed to measure the markers of oxidative stress in the following groups:

1. Twenty obese children without insulin resistance (ten males and ten females)
2. Twenty-two obese children with insulin resistance (ten males and twelve females)
3. Twenty-one non-diabetic children of normal weight

The results showed that glutathione peroxidase, an antioxidant enzyme, was lower, and nitrite/nitrate (a marker of oxidative stress) levels were higher in obese children with insulin resistance compared to the obese children without insulin resistance, as well as compared to non-diabetic children (Ozgen et al. 2012). Thus, increased oxidative stress occurs in children with insulin resistance, which can contribute to the development of type 2 diabetes.

Another clinical study involving twenty non-obese sedentary males and twenty females demonstrated that over-feeding induced insulin resistance by increasing oxidative stress (Samocha-Bonet et al. 2012). In order to demonstrate the role of oxidative stress in diabetes-related heart-disease complications, a clinical study was performed to measure the markers of oxidative stress in thirty-five diabetic post-menopausal females with heart-disease complications, and thirty-five age-matched type 2 diabetic post-menopausal females without heart-disease complications. All diabetic patients had high levels of glucose. However, the markers of oxidative stress such as increased levels of malondialdehyde (MDA) and decreased levels of glutathione, glutathione peroxidase, and superoxide dismutase (SOD) were present in diabetic patients with heart-disease complications, but not in diabetic patients without heart-disease complications (Kumawat et al. 2012).

Lymphocyte dysfunction makes patients with type 2 diabetes more susceptible to infection. It was demonstrated that lymphocyte dysfunction in patients with type 2 diabetes may be due to the damage to mitochondrial DNA by free radicals (Khan et al. 2011).

METABOLIC SYNDROME

Increased oxidative stress also occurs in individuals with metabolic syndrome. Increased levels of insulin and impaired glycemic control were associated with higher levels of oxidized low density lipids (LDL) in patients with metabolic syndrome (Holvoet 2008). This suggests that increased oxidative stress occurs in individuals with metabolic syndrome.

In a clinical study involving forty-three individuals with metabolic syndrome without type 2 diabetes and thirty-three healthy individuals without metabolic syndrome, the blood levels of markers of oxidative stress were determined. The results showed that the release of free radicals (superoxide anion) from monocytes was enhanced in individuals with metabolic syndrome compared to individuals without it. The expression of NADPH oxidase on the cell membrane was also increased in subjects with metabolic syndrome compared to those without metabolic syndrome. Furthermore, the levels of nuclear factor erythroid 2-related factor (involved in cellular antioxidant defense) decreased in monocytes obtained from the individuals with metabolic syndrome compared to those without metabolic syndrome.

The plasma levels of nitrotyrosine (an amino acid damaged by free radicals derived from nitrogen) and oxidized LDL cholesterol (markers of increased oxidative stress) were elevated in patients with metabolic syndrome compared to those without metabolic syndrome (Jialal et al. 2012).

A survey of data from the National Health and Nutrition Survey (NHANES) 2001–2006 revealed that the incidence of metabolic syndrome among adolescents between the ages of twelve and nineteen was 7 percent for boys and 3 percent for girls. Lower levels of carotenoids were associated with insulin resistance and higher levels of C-reactive protein in patients with metabolic syndrome. Vitamin C levels were also lower in patients with metabolic syndrome than those without it. Vitamin E levels in plasma were found to have no association with metabolic syndrome (Beydoun et al. 2012).

Adiponectin is a protein hormone secreted by fat cells. It helps to regulate the plasma level of glucose and breaks down fatty acids. The level of adiponectin decreased, whereas the level of MDA increased, in patients with metabolic syndrome (Sankhla et al. 2012).

A series of recent studies also support the role of increased oxidative stress in the development and progression of metabolic syndrome (Aroor et al. 2012; Pietropaoli et al. 2012; Venturini et al. 2012).

Next we will look at inflammation and see how it relates to the development of diabetes.

INFLAMMATION

Inflammation in Latin is referred to as *inflammare,* which means "setting on fire." The primary features of inflammation at affected sites include redness, swelling, warmth, and varying degrees of pain. These characteristics of inflammation were first recognized by the renowned Roman medical scholar, Aulus Cornelius Celsus (circa 25 BCE–50 CE).

The cell injury that results in inflammation can be caused by physical agents such as radiation, chemical toxins, mechanical trauma, or infection. Inflammation is divided into two categories, acute and chronic. Acute inflammation occurs following cellular injury or an infection by microorganisms. The period of acute inflammation is typically relatively short, lasting from a few minutes to a few days. Acute inflammation soon after an injury can help to heal the injury when tissue damage is not severe. If the tissue damage is extensive, however, acute inflammatory reactions may continue. The toxic products released during acute inflammation may contribute to organ failure and, eventually, to death.

Chronic inflammation occurs following *persistent* cellular injury and infection. The period of chronic inflammation is relatively long and can last as long as the injury or infection exists. The main features of chronic inflammation are the presence of immune cells such as lymphocytes and macrophages, which participate in inflammatory reactions. Chronic inflammation is associated with most chronic diseases, including heart disease and diabetes.

Inflammation is generally considered a protective response; however, it can act as a double-edged sword. It is needed to kill harmful invading organisms and for the removal of cellular debris in order to facilitate the recovery process at the site of injury, but inflammation can also damage normal tissue by releasing a number of toxic chemicals.

This is a highly complex biological response that is tightly regulated and automatically turned off after the completion of the recovery process. During the healing process, the injured tissue is replaced by regeneration of the original cell type, by filling of the injured site with fibroblastic tissue (scarring), or, most commonly, by a combination of both processes. If the damage is not repaired, however, a chronic inflammatory response is set in motion.

Features and Markers of Chronic Inflammation

Features of chronic inflammation include the proliferation of blood vessels, fibrosis (the increased proliferation of fibroblasts), tissue necrosis (cell death), and as mentioned above, the presence of an increased number of lymphocytes and macrophages.

As regards markers of inflammation, during chronic inflammation several potentially damaging agents are released. We will examine the prevalence of them in humans and in animals as well.

Markers of chronic inflammation include the following:

- Adhesion molecules
- Complement proteins
- C-reactive proteins (CRP)
- Cytokines (pro-inflammatory and anti-inflammatory)
- Eicosanoids (arachidonic acid metabolites)
- Reactive oxygen species (ROS; free radicals derived from oxygen)

Let's now look at these damaging agents a little more closely.

Adhesion Molecules

Adhesion molecules are sticky cell surface proteins that facilitate binding and communication between cells. They are called cell adhesion molecules (CAMs). Although CAMs are essential for the normal development and function of blood vessels, elevated levels have been implicated in the development and progression of diabetes. They also participate in inflammatory processes and wound-healing and play a significant role in the development and progression of heart disease. There are three major types of CAMs: integrins, selectins, and immunoglobulin molecules. The functions of these adhesion molecules are briefly described here.

Integrins: Integrins are a large group of glycoproteins with diverse biological functions. They are composed of two sub-units: integrin-alpha and integrin-beta. They facilitate the cell-cell binding and the adhesion of cells to an extracellular protein matrix such as collagen and fibronectin (Hillis and Flapan 1998). They also influence platelet aggregation, which may increase the risk of heart disease.

Selectins: Selectins bind with carbohydrates rather than proteins. There are three major forms of selectins. Selectins derived from lymphocytes are called selectin-L, those derived from platelets are called selectin-P, and those derived from endothelial cells are called selectin-E. The main function of selectin is to recruit leukocytes (white blood cells) to endothelium cells during inflammation, which contributes to the development and progression of diabetes by impairing blood-vessel function.

Immunoglobulin molecules: There are three major forms of immunoglobulin molecules: intercellular adhesion molecules (ICAM-1, -2, and -3), vascular cell adhesion molecule-1 (VCAM-1), and platelet endothelial cell adhesion molecule-1 (PECAM-1). ICAM-1 and -2 are found in endothelial cells, lymphocytes, and leukocytes circulating in the blood. They help in the migration of leukocytes at the site of inflammation in endothelial cells. VCAM-1 is found in large amounts on the surface of endothelial cells activated by pro-inflammatory cytokines (Golias et al. 2007). This helps to insure that leukocytes remain bound to the walls of blood vessels. PECAM-1 regulates the migration of leukocytes between endothelial cells and promotes the release of protease enzymes from the neutrophils.

Complement Proteins

Complement proteins are essential for the proper functioning of the immune system. The blood contains more than thirty complement proteins, including their degradation products, which help immune cells fight infection in the following ways:

1. They enhance the phagocytic activity (the engulfing ability) of macrophages.
2. They attract macrophages and neutrophils by inducing inflammation in order to kill invading bacteria or viruses.
3. They rupture the membrane of invading infectious agents such as bacteria and viruses.

The complement proteins are made primarily in liver cells, but cells of other organs such as the heart, the intestine, and the immune system (macrophages and monocytes) also make these proteins. Complement proteins are numbered C-1 through C-9, each of which has a complex mechanism of action on the cells. Although activation of complement proteins is essential for protecting the host against infectious agents such as bacteria and viruses, over-activation of these proteins may cause inflammation, which releases toxic products, thereby potentially increasing the risk of the development of atherosclerosis and heart disease. That activated complement proteins have a harmful effect on the heart is supported by the fact that an inhibition of activation of complement proteins reduced damage to the heart (Aukrust et al. 2001).

The activation of complement proteins plays an important role in the development of atherosclerosis (Malik et al. 2010).

Elevated levels of the complement protein C-3 has been found in heart disease (Onat et al. 2010); therefore, it can be used as a marker of heart disease.

Agents that activate complement proteins include the following:

1. Environmental allergens
2. Infectious agents (bacteria and viruses)
3. Antibodies

Although activation of complement proteins is essential for protecting the host against infectious agents such as bacteria and viruses, over-activation of these proteins may cause inflammation and thereby increase the risk of diabetes, as well as atherosclerosis and heart disease. Thus reducing the over-activation of complement proteins may reduce the risk of developing these diseases.

C-Reactive Proteins (CRP)

CRP in the blood is considered one of the markers of chronic inflammation. Extensive studies indicate that increased levels of CRP are associated with an increased risk of developing diabetes. In patients with metabolic syndrome, IL-18 was a strong predictor of the disease, whereas in patients without metabolic syndrome, CRP appears to be a strong predictor of diabetes. Elevated levels of fasting glucose increased the predictive value of IL-18 in patients with diabetes and metabolic syndrome (Troseid et al. 2009).

Cytokines (pro-inflammatory and anti-inflammatory)

A cytokine is a small protein that is made by one cell and acts on another. They are released during both acute and chronic inflammation. They are produced primarily by activated immune cells such as lymphocytes and macrophages. There are two types of cytokines: pro-inflammatory and anti-inflammatory. A complex network of cytokines maintains a balance between the effects of pro-inflammatory cytokines and anti-inflammatory cytokines. If this balance is altered in favor of pro-inflammatory cytokines, chronic diseases such as heart disease and diabetes may develop. Examples of pro-inflammatory cytokines include interleukin-1 (IL-1), interleukin-6 (IL-6), interleukin-8 (IL-8), interleukin-15 (IL-15), interleukin-16 (IL-16), interleukin-17 (IL-17), and interleukin-18 (IL-18), tumor necrosis factor-alpha, TGF-beta, and interferon-gamma. These pro-inflammatory cytokines are damaging to the cells of the body.

Anti-inflammatory cytokines, on the other hand, include interleukin-4 (IL-4), interleukin-10 (IL-10), interleukin-11 (IL-11), and interleukin-13 (IL-13). These cytokines, which help to heal damaged tissue, are released in response to an injury by infection, increased oxidative damage to the cells, or by physical injury to the cells.

Eicosanoids (arachiodonic acid metabolites)

During inflammation, arachidonic acid (AA) metabolites (also called eicosanoids) are released. Eicosanoids include prostaglandins (PGs), thromboxanes, leukotrienes, and lipoxins. There are different forms of PGs and thromboxanes. Some of them dilate blood vessels and prevent platelet aggregation, whereas others cause an aggregation of platelets. For example, prostacyclin (PGI2) is a potent dilator of blood vessels and reduces platelet aggregation. In contrast, thromboxane A2 (TXA2) causes an aggregation of platelets. Aspirin reduces the formation of both PGs and thromboxanes by inhibiting the enzyme cyclooxygenase (COX).

Neoptrin

Neoptrin is a chemical substance made in macrophages following stimulation by the cytokine interferon-gamma. It is a marker of inflammation, and high blood levels of it are associated with the increased production of reactive oxygen species.

These results further support the idea that increased chronic inflammation plays a role in the development and progression of diabetes.

Inflammation Markers in Diabetic Animals

Inflammatory molecules and their transcriptional factor, NF-kappa B, appear to play an important role in diabetes-induced heart disease. In diabetic mice, increased NF-kappa B activity was associated with enhanced oxidative stress. Administration of pyrrolidine dithiocarbamates (PDTC), a NF-kappaB inhibitor, reduced oxidative stress and improved mitochondrial dysfunction in these same mice (Mariappan et al. 2010).

In a rat model of diabetes, elevated levels of IL-1 beta in islet cells promotes cytokine and chemokine expression, leading to the recruitment of immune cells. Therefore, IL-1 beta may not produce a direct toxic effect on islet beta-cells, but may induce tissue inflammation causing beta-cell death and insulin resistance in type 2 diabetes (Ehses et al. 2009).

In mice models of type 2 diabetes, the interaction between NF-kappa B and TNF-alpha signaling induced the activation of IKK-beta, which amplified oxidative stress, leading to endothelial dysfunction (Yang et al. 2009).

It has also been reported that increased expression of p53 in mouse adipose tissue contributes to insulin resistance caused by enhanced inflammatory responses (Minamino et al. 2009).

Inflammation Markers in Diabetic Humans

The histology of islet cells from patients with type 2 diabetes exhibited the presence of inflammatory products such as cytokines, as well as immune cell infiltration and fibrosis (Donath et al. 2008).

Inflammatory molecules such as IL-beta, interferon-gamma (IFN-gamma), and TNF-alpha contribute to beta-cell death by activating NF-kappaB activity. This was confirmed by the fact that blocking NF-kappaB activation protected beta-cells against IL-beta + IFN-gamma or TNF-alpha + IFN-gamma-induced apoptosis (Ortis et al. 2008). Thus, activation of NF-kappaB activity appears to be an important event in the progressive loss of beta-cells from the pancreas in diabetes.

In obesity, adipose tissue is infiltrated by macrophages that release excessive amounts of inflammatory molecules, including TNF-alpha and IL-6, which contribute to insulin resistance in patients with type 2 diabetes (Bastard et al. 2006; Heilbronn and Campbell 2008).

In a clinical study involving ten individuals of normal weight and eight obese subjects, the effects of a high-fat and high-carbohydrate meal on markers of oxidative stress and chronic inflammation after an overnight fast were evaluated. The results showed that high-fat, high-carbohydrate meals induced significantly more prolonged and greater oxidative stress and inflammation in the obese subjects compared to individuals of normal weight (Patel et al. 2007). A persistent increase in oxidative stress and chronic inflammation may increase the risk of developing insulin resistance, diabetes, and heart disease.

The effects of the infusion of high-glucose doses on markers of inflammation were tested in twenty-two men with type 1 diabetes and thirteen age-matched individuals without type 1 diabetes. The results showed that increased plasma glucose levels enhanced the levels of markers of chronic inflammation IL-6 and tumor necrosis factor-alpha (TNF-alpha) (Gordin et al. 2008). This suggests that acute hyperglycemia increases the levels of markers of inflammation in patients with type 1 diabetes.

In a clinical study involving seventy-six patients with type 1 diabetes and thirty healthy (non-diabetic) patients, the levels of markers of pro-inflammatory cytokines were determined. The results showed that the plasma levels of CRP, TNF-alpha, and IL-6 were higher in patients with type 1 diabetes than in non-diabetic patients (Mitrovic et al. 2011).

It was demonstrated that patients with type 2 diabetes and insulin resistance and those with abnormal lipid levels had higher levels of IL-12 compared to non-diabetic patients (Mishra et al. 2011).

The levels of vascular cell adhesion molecule-1 (VCAM-1) and intercellular adhesion molecule-1 (ICAM-1) were also elevated in patients with diabetes compared to normal subjects. The levels of CRP and reactive oxygen species were higher in patients with metabolic syndrome (one hundred twenty-three patients) than in those individuals without metabolic syndrome (three hundred thirty-four subjects) (Kotani and Sakane 2012).

CONCLUDING REMARKS

Free radicals are highly damaging chemicals that are produced in the human body. They are generated during the use of oxygen, in the course of bacterial or viral infection, and in the context of the normal metabolism of certain compounds. There are several types of free radicals: some are derived from oxygen whereas others are derived from nitrogen. Oxidative stress refers to a condition in the body in which high levels of free radicals are produced, causing damage to the cells. Increased oxidative stress may be one of the important factors involved in an elevated risk of developing diabetes.

Additionally, cell injury caused by physical agents—such as radiation, free radicals, chemical toxins, mechanical trauma, or infection—initiates an important biological event called inflammation. Inflammation is generally considered a protective response, for while it is needed to kill invading harmful organisms, and for the removal of cellular debris in order to facilitate the recovery process at the site of injury, it can also damage normal tissue by releasing a number of toxic chemicals.

The studies presented in this chapter show that increased oxidative stress and chronic inflammation play an important role in the development and progression of type 1 diabetes, type 2 diabetes, and metabolic syndrome. Even obese individuals who are at a high risk of developing type 2 diabetes have increased oxidative stress. Therefore, agents that decrease levels of oxidative stress and chronic inflammation may reduce the risk of the development and progression of these diseases. Among various preventive agents, antioxidants, which are non-toxic and which decrease both free radicals and chronic inflammation, help to reduce the development and progression of diabetes.

In the following chapters we will present a general overview of antioxidants and discuss why they are essential for optimal health. Subsequently, we will discuss the role of antioxidants specifically as it pertains to diabetes prevention, and in this, we will present the results of numerous studies to illustrate what has been discovered to date.

3 The Antioxidant Defense System

Vitamins and Micronutrients

In this chapter* we will more fully explore the antioxidant defense system and the roles that antioxidants play in safeguarding the body's health and well-being. We will also detail the history of antioxidants, their actions and sources, and discuss their defining properties, commercial availability, and other important information about them and their use. Let's now take a closer look at the antioxidant defense system of the human body and expand our understanding of the functions of these very important substances.

THE ANTIOXIDANT DEFENSE SYSTEM AND ITS FUNCTIONS

The antioxidant defense system in humans can be divided into two groups: (a) endogenous antioxidants that are made in the body and (b) exogenous antioxidants that are not made in the body but consumed through diet (standard dietary antioxidants).

Endogenous antioxidants include antioxidant enzymes such as superoxide dismutase (SOD), catalase, and glutathione peroxidase. They

---

*Much of the material in this chapter is derived from *Fighting Cancer with Vitamins and Antioxidants,* Prasad and Prasad, 2011.

also include compounds such as glutathione, alpha-lipoic acid, coenzyme Q10, L-carnitine, and melatonin. (Antioxidant enzymes are not effective when taken orally because they are degraded in the intestinal tract.)

Exogenous antioxidants (standard dietary antioxidants) that are commonly used in a multivitamin preparation include vitamins A, C, D (in the form of D-3), E, and beta-carotene. Exogenous antioxidants derived from herbal, fruit, and vegetable sources include resveratrol, curcumin, cinnamon extract, and ginseng extract, although they are not always added to a multivitamin preparation. However, in the case of diabetes, some herbal antioxidants such as curcumin, cinnamon bark, and milk thistle may be added because they are capable of producing beneficial effects that are not related to the destruction of free radicals alone. (We will discuss the addition of these antioxidants to a multivitamin formulation in greater detail later in the book.)

Why are free radicals so important, and what *exactly* do they do for us? Many people have traditionally believed that antioxidants have only one function—to neutralize free radicals—but in view of recent advances in antioxidant research, this belief is incorrect. The actions of antioxidants on cells and tissues are varied and complex. In addition to neutralizing free radicals, antioxidants reduce inflammation, stimulate immune function, participate in several biological processes, and regulate the genetic activity involved in proliferation, growth, and differentiation (converting immature cells to adult-type cells). Each antioxidant has some unique functions that cannot be replicated by the others.

Summary of Known Actions of Antioxidants

1. Scavenge free radicals
2. Decrease markers of pro-inflammatory cytokines
3. Alter gene expression profiles
4. Alter protein kinase activity

> 5. Prevent release and toxicity of excessive amounts of glutamate
> 6. Participate in several biological processes
> 7. Induce cell differentiation (maturation) in normal cells during development
> 8. Increase immune function

THE HISTORY AND
ACTIONS OF MAJOR ANTIOXIDANTS

Vitamin A

Night blindness, which we now know is caused by vitamin A deficiency, existed for centuries before the discovery of vitamin A. As early as approximately 1500 BCE, Egyptians knew how to cure this condition. Roman soldiers suffering from night blindness would travel to Egypt to receive liver extract, which cured it. (Today, it is well established that liver is the richest source of vitamin A.)

In 1912 Dr. Elmer McCollum of the University of Wisconsin discovered vitamin A in butter. It was initially called fat-soluble A. The structure of vitamin A was determined in 1930, and it was first synthesized in the laboratory in 1947.

In addition to maintaining vision, vitamin A plays an important role in stimulating immune function, regulating gene activity, and proper embryonic development, as well as playing a role in reproduction, bone metabolism, and enhancing skin health.

The B Vitamins

All of the B vitamins were discovered during the years 1912–1934. In the year 1912, the Polish-born biochemist Dr. C. Funk isolated their active substances from the rice husks of unpolished rice, which prevented the disease beriberi. This disease affects many parts of the body including muscle tissue, the heart, the nervous system, and the digestive system. Dr. Funk named the substances he discovered vita-mines, because he thought they were "amines" derived from ammonia. In 1920, the *e* was dropped when it became known that not all vita-mins are "amines." Today there are many different vitamins within the vitamin B family.

Carotenoids

There are several types of carotenoids in plants, fruits, and vegetables; they are known to protect against damage produced by ultraviolet light and by free radicals generated from ionizing radiation (like X-rays) and other chemicals. In 1919, carotenoid pigments were isolated from yellow plants, and in 1930 it was found that some of the ingested carotenes were converted to vitamin A. This carotene was referred to as beta-carotene. Beta-carotene not only acts as a precursor of vitamin A, but it also has some effects that cannot be produced by vitamin A.

For example, beta-carotene increases the expression of the connexin gene that codes for a gap junction protein, which holds two normal cells together. (Vitamin A cannot produce such an effect.) In addition, beta-carotene is a more effective destroyer of free radicals in high-oxygen pressure (high concentration of oxygen) in the body tissues than vita-min A.

Vitamin C

Scurvy, we know today, is caused by vitamin C deficiency; however, its symptoms were known to the Egyptians as early as 1500 BCE. In the fifth century, Hippocrates described the symptoms of scurvy, which include bleeding gums, hemorrhaging, and death. Native American Indians had a cure for scurvy that included drinking the extract of pine bark and needles (prepared like tea), but this cure remained limited to their own population for hundreds of years.

During the sea voyages of European explorers between the twelfth and sixteenth centuries, the epidemic of scurvy among sailors forced some of them to land in Canada, where native Indians gave them their concoction of pine bark and needles, thus curing their scurvy.

In 1536, Jacques Cartier, a French explorer, brought this formulation to France, but the medical establishment rejected it as fraud because it came from Native Americans.

By 1593, Sir Richard Hawkins recommended to his sailors that they eat oranges and lemons to reduce the risk of disease but it wasn't until 1770 that the British Navy began recommending that ships carry sufficient lime juice for all personnel. In 1928, Albert Szent-Györgyi, a Hungarian scientist, isolated hexuronic acid from the adrenal gland. This substance was vitamin C, and in 1932 it became the first vitamin to be made in the laboratory.

Vitamin C acts as an antioxidant and participates in several enzyme activities that are needed for the proper functioning of the organs. It helps in the formation of collagen, and it also takes part in the formation of interferon, a naturally occurring anti-viral agent. Additionally, it regenerates damaged vitamin E to an active form.

Vitamin D

Although the bone disease known as rickets may have existed in human populations for centuries, it was not until the year 1645 that English physician Dr. Daniel Whistler described its symptoms, which we now know are due to vitamin D deficiency. In 1922, Sir Edward Mellanby, while working on a cure for rickets, officially discovered vitamin D. It was later found to require sunlight for its formation in the body's skin cells. In 1930, the chemical structure of this vitamin was determined by a German scientist named Adolf Windaus. Vitamin D_3 is the most active form of vitamin D. It was chemically characterized in 1936, and was initially thought to be a steroid effective in the treatment of rickets.

Vitamin D is essential for bone formation, and regulates calcium and phosphorus levels in the blood. It also inhibits parathyroid hormone secretion from the parathyroid glands, and stimulates immune function by promoting phagocytosis.

Vitamin E

In 1922, Dr. Herbert Evans of the University of California, Berkeley, observed that rats reared exclusively on whole milk grew normally but were not fertile. Fertility was restored when they were fed additional wheat germ. However, it took another fourteen years, until 1936, before the active substance responsible for restoring fertility was isolated. Dr. Evans named it tocopherol, from the Greek word meaning "to bear offspring." The "ol" ending signifies its chemical status as an alcohol. Tocopherol is also called vitamin E.

Vitamin E acts as an antioxidant, regulates genetic activity, and relocates certain proteins from one compartment to another within the same cell. It helps to maintain skin health, reduces scarring, and acts as an anti-coagulant at very high doses. Vitamin E reduces inflammation, and stimulates immune function. Its derivative, vitamin E succinate, is considered the most effective form of vitamin E.

ENDOGENOUS ANTIOXIDANTS AND THEIR ACTIONS

Endogenous antioxidants, as we have learned, are made in the body. They include antioxidant enzymes and compounds, some of which are detailed below.

Catalase

The antioxidant enzyme catalase needs iron for its biological activity; it destroys hydrogen peroxide in cells.

Coenzyme Q10

In 1957, Dr. Fredrick Crane, working at the University of Wisconsin, isolated coenzyme Q10. One year later, at Merck Laboratories, Dr. O. E. Wolf, working under Dr. Karl Folkers, determined the structure of coenzyme Q10. It is a weak antioxidant, but is significant because it recycles vitamin E to an active form. Coenzyme Q10 is essential for generating energy within mitochondria, thereby generating energy for the cells of the human body.

The heart and the liver, which require the most energy, have the highest concentrations of coenzyme Q10 due to the large number of mitochondria found in these organs. Other organelles inside the cells that contain coenzyme Q10 include endoplasmic reticulum, peroxisomes, lysosomes, and the Golgi apparatus.

Glutathione

Glutathione is formed in the body from three amino acids: L-cysteine, L-glutamic acid, and L-glycine. It is present in all of the cells in a reduced or oxidized form, with the highest concentration of it found in the liver. In healthy cells, more than 90 percent of glutathione is present in the reduced form. The oxidized form of glutathione can be converted to the reduced form by the enzyme glutathione reductase; this reduced form acts as an antioxidant.

Glutathione is one of the most important antioxidants in that it protects cellular components inside of the cells. It is needed for the detoxification of toxins that are produced as by-products of normal metabolism, as well as certain exogenous toxins. Glutathione also participates in several enzyme activities and reduces inflammation.

Glutathione peroxidase

The antioxidant enzyme glutathione peroxidase requires selenium for its biological activity and is responsible for removing hydrogen peroxide.

L-carnitine

L-carnitine was originally found to be a growth factor for mealworms. It is synthesized from the amino acids lysine and methionine, primarily in the liver and the kidneys. It exists as L-carnitine, a biologically active form, and as D-carnitine, a biologically inactive form. Vitamin C is necessary for its synthesis.

Polyphenols

Polyphenols are a very numerous group of chemical substances found in plants; they are also referred to as phytochemicals. They are present in herbs, fruits, and vegetables. Examples of them include resveratrol (in grape skin and seed), curcumin (in the spice turmeric), ginseng extract, cinnamon extract, and garlic extract. Generally fat-soluble, they are absorbed from the intestinal tract and distributed in all of the tissues of the body. Resveratrol in particular has drawn a great deal of attention in recent years; it is found in grape skin and grape seed.

Other polyphenols include tannins, lignins, and flavonoids. The largest and the most widely studied polyphenols are flavonoids, which include quercetin, epicatechin, and oligomeric proanthocyanidins. The major sources of flavonoids include all citrus fruits, berries, ginkgo biloba, onions, parsley, tea, red wine, and dark chocolate. Over 5,000 naturally occurring flavonoids have been characterized from various plants. Flavonoids are poorly absorbed by the human intestinal tract. All flavonoids possess varying degrees of antioxidant activity.

Superoxide Dismutase (SOD)

The antioxidant enzyme SOD requires manganese, copper, or zinc for its biological activity. Manganese (Mn)-SOD is present in the mitochondria whereas copper (Cu)-SOD and zinc (Zn)-SOD are present in the cytoplasm and the nucleus of the cell. They can destroy free radicals and hydrogen peroxide.

EXOGENOUS ANTIOXIDANTS (STANDARD DIETARY ANTIOXIDANTS) AND THEIR SOURCES

Vitamins A, C, and E, as well as carotenoids and the mineral selenium, are exogenous antioxidants that are also referred to as "standard dietary antioxidants," because they are commonly consumed through diet or used in a multivitamin preparation. Other types of exogenous antioxidants include various kinds of polyphenols (referenced above) that are found in fruits, vegetables, and herbs, some of which are often added to a multivitamin preparation in small quantities.

The sources of some standard dietary antioxidants are described below.

Vitamin A

The richest source of vitamin A is liver (6.5 milligrams per 100 grams of liver) from beef, pork, chicken, turkey, and fish. Vitamin A exists as retinyl palmitate or retinyl acetate, which is converted into the retinol form in the body. Retinol is converted to retinoic acid in the cells. It has been determined that 1 IU (international unit) of vitamin A equals 0.3 micrograms of retinol. Vitamin A and its derivative retinoids in natural and synthetic forms are commercially available.

Carotenoids/Beta-Carotene

There are more than six hundred carotenoids in various plants, fruits, and vegetables. Among them, beta-carotene, alpha-carotene, lycopene, lutein, xanthophylls, zeaxanthin, and beta-cryptoxanthin are important. (We do not know much about many of the other carotenoids.) Beta-carotene, alpha-carotene, lycopene, and lutein have been studied extensively in laboratory experiments and in humans.

The richest sources of carotenoids are sweet potatoes, carrots, spinach, mango, cantaloupe, apricot, kale, broccoli, parsley, cilantro, pumpkins, winter squash, and fresh thyme. It has been determined that 1 IU (international unit) of vitamin A equals 0.6 micrograms of beta-carotene. One molecule of beta-carotene produces two molecules of vitamin A. Beta-carotene in its natural and synthetic forms is commercially available.

Vitamin C

The richest sources of vitamin C are fruits and vegetables. They include rose hip, red pepper, parsley, guava, kiwi fruit, broccoli, lychee, papaya, and strawberry. Each of these fruits or vegetables contains approximately 2,000 milligrams of vitamin C per 100 grams of fruit. Other sources of vitamin C include oranges, lemons, melon, garlic, cauliflower, grapefruit, raspberries, tangerines, passion fruit, spinach, and limes. They contain about 30 to 50 milligrams per 100 grams of fruit and vegetable. Vitamin C is sold commercially as L-ascorbic acid, calcium ascorbate, sodium ascorbate, and potassium ascorbate.

Vitamin E

The richest sources of vitamin E include wheat germ oil (215 milligrams per 100 of grams of oil), sunflower oil (56 milligrams per 100 grams of oil), olive oil (12 milligrams per 100 grams of oil), almond oil (39 milligrams per 100 grams of oil), hazelnut oil (26 milligrams per 100 grams of oil), walnut oil (20 milligrams per 100 grams of oil), and peanut oil (17 milligrams per 100 grams of oil). Sources for small amounts of vitamin E (0.1 to 2 milligrams per 100 grams) include kiwi fruit, fish, leafy vegetables, and whole grains. In the United States, fortified breakfast cereals are important sources of vitamin E.

At present, most of the natural form of vitamin E is extracted from vegetable oils, primarily soybean oil. Vitamin E exists in eight different forms: four tocopherols (alpha-, beta-, gamma-, and delta-tocopherol), and four tocotrienols (alpha-, beta-, gamma-, and delta-tocotrienol). Of these, alpha-tocopherol has the most biological activity. Vitamin E can exist in the natural form commonly indicated as "d," whereas the synthetic form is referred to as "dl." The stable esterified form of vitamin E is available as alpha-tocopheryl acetate, alpha-tocopheryl succinate, and alpha-tocopheryl nicotinate. The activity of vitamin E is generally expressed in international units (IU). It is determined that 1 IU of vitamin E equals 0.66 milligrams of d-alpha-tocopherol, and 1 IU of racemic mixture (dl-form) equals 0.45 milligrams of d-alpha-tocopherol.

PROPERTIES
OF ANTIOXIDANTS

Solubility

Lipid-soluble antioxidants include vitamin A, vitamin E, carotenoids, coenzyme Q10, and L-carnitine. These fat-soluble vitamins should be taken with meals, so that they can be more readily absorbed. Water-soluble antioxidants include vitamin C, glutathione, and alpha-lipoic acid.

Toxicity

High doses of antioxidants have been consumed by the U.S. population for decades without significant toxicity. However, they may be harmful for some individuals when consumed daily for a long period of time.

For example, vitamin A at doses of 10,000 IU or more per day can cause birth defects in pregnant women, and beta-carotene at doses of 50 milligrams or more can produce bronzing of the skin that is reversible on discontinuation. Vitamin C as ascorbic acid at high doses (10 grams or more per day) can cause diarrhea in some individuals. Vitamin E at high doses (2,000 IU or more per day) can induce clotting defects after long-term consumption. Vitamin B_6 at high doses (50 milligrams or more per day) can produce peripheral neuropathy (numbness of the extremities), and selenium at doses of 400 micrograms or more per day can cause skin and liver toxicity after long-term consumption.

Coenzyme Q10 has no known toxicity; recommended daily doses of it are 300–400 milligrams. N-acetylcysteine doses of 250–1500 milligrams and alpha-lipoic acid doses of 600 milligrams are used in humans, without toxicity.

We will look at the toxicity of antioxidants in greater detail in the following chapter.

COMMERCIALLY AVAILABLE ANTIOXIDANTS AND THEIR DISTRIBUTION IN THE BODY

Next we will examine the commercial availability of some antioxidants, and although we do include some recommendations here, later in the book we will cover these recommendations more comprehensively.

Vitamin A

Vitamin A is sold commercially as retinyl palmitate, retinyl acetate, and retinoic acid and its analogues. Retinyl acetate or retinyl palmitate (a stable form sold commercially) is converted to retinol (a form present in the body) in the intestine before absorption. Retinol is then converted to retinoic acid in the cells. Retinoic acid performs all the functions of vitamin A except that of maintaining vision. Retinoic acid and its derivatives are used in laboratory studies because they are readily soluble in fat and thus enter cells easily. Vitamin A in blood takes the form of retinol and is stored in the liver as retinyl palmitate. Vitamin A exists as a protein-bound molecule. The vitamin A product retinoic acid is stored in all body tissues. As noted previously, vitamin A is a fat-soluble antioxidant.

Carotenoids/Beta-carotene

Beta-carotene is one of more than 600 carotenoids found in fruits, vegetables, and other plants. It is also commercially available in natural or synthetic forms. Laboratory experiments have demonstrated that the natural form of beta-carotene is more effective in reducing the risk of cancer than the synthetic form. Preparations of natural carotenoids contain primarily beta-carotene; however, other types of carotenoids are also present. Synthetic preparations of beta-carotene contain unknown impurities, the toxicity of which remains uncertain. A portion of ingested beta-carotene is converted to retinol (vitamin A) in the intestinal tract before absorption, and the remainder is distributed in the blood and tissues of the body. About twenty other carotenoids, including products of a variety of ingested carotenoids, also enter the blood and tissues. One molecule of beta-carotene forms two molecules of vitamin A.

In humans, the conversion of beta-carotene to vitamin A does not occur if the body has sufficient amounts of vitamin A. Beta carotene is primarily stored in the eyes and fatty tissue. Other carotenoids such as lycopene accumulate in the prostate more than in other organs, whereas lutein accumulates in the eyes more than other organs. Synthetic forms of lycopene and lutein are not commercially available. All carotenoids are considered fat-soluble antioxidants, which should be taken with meals in order that they are more readily absorbed.

Vitamin C

Vitamin C is commercially sold as ascorbic acid, sodium ascorbate (1 gram of this type of vitamin C contains 124 milligrams of sodium), magnesium ascorbate, calcium ascorbate, and time-release capsules containing ascorbic acid and vitamin C-ester. It is present in all the cells of the body. Vitamin C enters the blood as ascorbic acid, which can be converted to dehydroascorbic acid that can be re-converted to ascorbic acid.

All mammals make vitamin C except guinea pigs and humans. An adult goat makes about 13 grams of vitamin C every day. Vitamin C can recycle the non-antioxidant form of vitamin E (the oxidized form of vitamin E) to an antioxidant form. Ascorbic acid supplements at high doses can cause an upset stomach in some people. Sodium ascorbate at high doses may increase the concentration of sodium in the urine, which can lead to chronic irritation in the bladder. It should be noted that time-release capsules of vitamin C contain additional synthetic chemicals. Vitamin C-ester cannot function as vitamin C until the enzyme esterase removes the ester. For these reasons, we recommend calcium ascorbate, which is buffered and is unlikely to produce stomach upset. As we have learned, all forms of vitamin C are water-soluble.

Vitamin E

Vitamin E is a term used for all tocopherols and tocotrienols possessing the biological activity of alpha-tocopherol. Both tocopherol and tocotrienol have alpha (α), beta (β), gamma (γ), and delta (δ) forms. Alpha-tocopherol has the highest antioxidant activity, followed by beta-, gamma-, and delta-tocopherol. In recent years, research on tocotrienols has also revealed some important biological functions. Synthetic vitamin E is referred to as the dl form; the natural form is termed the d form. Vitamin E is commercially sold as d- or dl-tocopherol, alpha-tocopheryl acetate, or alpha-tocopheryl succinate (vitamin E succinate). Alpha-tocopheryl acetate and vitamin E succinate forms of vitamin E are more stable than alpha-tocopherol. Alpha-tocopherol, alpha-tocopheryl acetate, and vitamin E succinate have been widely used in laboratory and clinical studies. It has been presumed that alpha-tocopheryl acetate and vitamin E succinate are converted to alpha-tocopherol in the intestinal tract before absorption.

This assumption may be true as long as the stores of alpha-tocopherol in the body are not completely full; however, if they are full, a portion of vitamin E succinate can be absorbed as vitamin E succinate. Therefore, it is not necessary that all vitamin E succinate be converted to alpha-tocopherol before absorption. Vitamin E succinate enters the cells more easily than alpha-tocopherol because of its greater solubility. In addition, vitamin E succinate has some unique functions that cannot be produced by alpha-tocopherol.

Vitamin E succinate is now considered the most effective form of vitamin E in inhibiting the growth of cancer cells, but it cannot act as an antioxidant until converted to alpha-tocopherol. Laboratory experiments have shown that the solvents of some water-soluble preparations of vitamin E are toxic and should be avoided. Alpha-tocopherol is located primarily in the membranous structures of the cells.

Alpha-lipoic Acid

Alpha-lipoic acid is commercially available and should be added to a multivitamin preparation for the following reasons. It is a more potent antioxidant than vitamin C or vitamin E. It is soluble in both water and lipid; therefore, it protects cellular membranes as well as water-soluble compounds. It regenerates tissue levels of vitamin C and vitamin E and markedly elevates glutathione levels in cells. Alpha-lipoic acid participates in several enzyme activities.

Coenzyme Q10

Coenzyme Q10 is sold commercially as time-release capsules or simply as coenzyme Q10. A comparative study regarding the efficacy of time-release and the regular forms of coenzyme Q10 has not been made. We recommend a regular form of coenzyme Q10. This supplement is fat-soluble.

Glutathione

Glutathione is sold commercially for oral consumption; however, this antioxidant is totally destroyed in the intestine. Therefore, an oral administration of glutathione would not increase the level of glutathione in the cells and therefore will not produce any beneficial effect in the body.

L-carnitine

L-carnitine is made in the body, but we can also obtain it from the diet. The highest concentration of L-carnitine is found in red meat (95 milligrams per 3.0 ounces of meat). In contrast, chicken breast has only 3.9 milligrams per 3.5 ounces. L-carnitine is present in all of the cells of the body.

Melatonin

Melatonin is a naturally occurring hormone produced primarily by the pineal gland in the brain. It is also produced by the retina, lens, and gastrointestinal tract. Melatonin is formed from the amino acid tryptophan. Melatonin is also produced by various plants such as rice. It is readily absorbed from the intestinal tract; however, 50 percent of it is routinely removed from the plasma in thirty-five to fifty minutes.

Melatonin plays an important role in sleep in that it regulates circadian rhythms through its receptor. It also acts as an antioxidant, reduces inflammation, and stimulates immune function. Unlike other antioxidants, damaged melatonin cannot be regenerated by other antioxidants.

N-acetylcysteine (NAC)

N-acetylcysteine (NAC) is not made in the body, but in the laboratory from the amino acid cysteine, which is used to make glutathione in the body. NAC is not destroyed in the small intestine when consumed orally, and thus can be taken as a supplement. In the body, n-acetyl is removed from NAC by the enzyme esterase, and then cysteine is used to make glutathione. Alpha-lipoic acid also increases the level of glutathione by a mechanism that is different from NAC, and is present in all cells. This function is important because orally administered glutathione is totally destroyed in the small intestine. At high doses, n-acetylcysteine binds with metals and removes them from the body. For these reasons, it is beneficial to include NAC in a multivitamin preparation.

NADH (the reduced form of nicotinamide adenine dinucleotide)

Like L-carnitine, nicotinamide adenine dinucleotide (NAD+) and NADH are present in all of the cells of our body. NAD+ is an oxidizing agent; therefore, it can act as a pro-oxidant, whereas NADH can act as an antioxidant. NAD+ accepts electrons from other molecules and is reduced to the form NADH, which can recycle oxidized vitamin E to the reduced form, which can then act as an antioxidant. NADH is essential for mitochondria to generate energy and is water-soluble.

Polyphenols

Polyphenols are important antioxidants but they do not produce any unique biological effects that cannot be produced by standard dietary and endogenous antioxidants. While these agents are commercially available, the addition of one or more of these antioxidants to a multivitamin preparation is not necessary. They should be consumed through the diet regularly.

HOW TO STORE ANTIOXIDANTS

Vitamin A
Vitamin A as retinyl palmitate or retinyl acetate in solid form is stable at room temperature for a few years. The solid form of retinol or retinoic acid is not stable at room temperature; therefore, it can be stored at 4°C (in the refrigerator) for several months. A solution of retinoic acid is stable at 4° C, stored away from light, for several weeks.

Carotenoids
Most commercially sold carotenoids in solid form can be stored at room temperature and away from light for a few years. They should not be stored in solution, because they degrade within a few days, even if they are stored in a colder environment, away from light.

Vitamin C
Vitamin C should not be stored in liquid form because the liquid form is easily destroyed within a few days. Crystal or tablet forms of vitamin C can be kept at room temperature, away from light, for a few years.

Vitamin E
Alpha-tocopherol is relatively unstable at room temperature in comparison to alpha-tocopheryl acetate and alpha-tocopheryl succinate. Alpha tocopherol can be stored at 4°C for several weeks, but alpha-tocopheryl acetate and alpha-tocopheryl succinate can be stored at room temperature for a few years. A solution of alpha-tocopheryl succinate is stable for several months at 4°C, if kept away from light.

Coenzyme Q10 and NADH

These antioxidants in solid forms are stable at room temperature, away from light, for a few years. The solutions of these antioxidants are stable at 4°C, away from light, for several months.

Glutathione, N-acetylcysteine, and Alpha-lipoic Acid

Solid forms of glutathione, n-acetylcysteine, and alpha-lipoic acid are stable at room temperature, away from light, for a few years. The solutions of these antioxidants are stable at 4°C, away from light, for several months.

Melatonin

The powder form of melatonin is stable at room temperature for a year or more.

Polyphenols

Polyphenols are stable and can be stored in solid form at room temperature, away from light, for a few years.

CAN ANTIOXIDANTS BE DESTROYED DURING COOKING?

Some antioxidants are destroyed during cooking, some are not, and others are partially degraded. We will explore this very important feature next.

Vitamin A

Of all the vitamins, vitamin A appears to be the most sensitive to heat. Routine cooking does not destroy it significantly, but slow heating for a longer period of time may reduce its potency. The canning preparation of fruits and vegetables containing vitamin A may also diminish its potency. Prolonged cold storage may diminish it as well.

The vitamin A content of fortified milk powder substantially declines after two years.

Carotenoids

Most carotenoids, especially beta-carotene, lutein and lycopene, are not destroyed during cooking. In fact, their bioavailability improves when they are derived from a cooked or extracted preparation (such as lycopene from tomato sauce). These carotenoids are extracted during cooking, and thus, are easily absorbed from the intestine.

Vitamin E

Food processing, frying, and freezing destroy vitamin E. The vitamin E content of fortified milk powder is unaffected over a two-year period.

Coenzyme Q10 and NADH

Coenzyme Q10 and NADH can be partially degraded during cooking.

Glutathione, N-acetylcysteine, and Alpha-lipoic acid

Glutathione, n-acetylcysteine, and alpha-lipoic acid can be partially destroyed during cooking.

Polyphenols

Polyphenols are not destroyed during cooking.

CONCLUDING REMARKS

In this chapter we learned the various functions that antioxidants play in the maintenance of optimal health, and how essential they are in helping to keep disease at bay. Some antioxidants are made in the body, whereas others are consumed through a diet containing fruits and vegetables. Both endogenous and exogenous (standard dietary antioxidants) are important for optimal health and chronic disease prevention. The inclusion of different types of antioxidants is also important because some have unique functions that are not replicated by others. It is also important to understand their potential toxicity, as well as their other properties.

In the next chapter we will examine our antioxidant needs more closely, and discuss how to best insure that these needs are met.

4 Why We Need Supplementary Micronutrients

Many harmful chemicals are generated during the digestion of food. These include mutagens that alter genetic activity, and carcinogens. Non-vegetarians form these toxic substances more than vegetarians do,* a portion of which are absorbed from the gastrointestinal tract, thereby potentially increasing the risk of chronic disease over a long period of time. Maintaining an adequate amount of micronutrients in the body, including antioxidants, is vital, given that in so doing, the formation of these toxic chemicals can be reduced.

The RDA (Recommended Dietary Allowances) is now referred to as DRI (Dietary Reference Intakes); however, food labels continue to use the designation of RDA, not DRI. The RDA/DRI has been established for each micronutrient (which includes antioxidants, as we know). These values are considered sufficient for preventing deficiencies and for enhancing growth and development. However, these values may not be sufficient for optimal health and chronic disease prevention or treatment. That is to say that most standard antioxidants may not be obtainable in adequate amounts from one's diet alone (though polyphenols of various kinds can adequately be obtained from the diet).

---

*The consumption of organic food does not affect the amounts of toxins formed during the digestive process.

This entire matter is complicated by the fact that only about 10 percent of ingested water-soluble or fat-soluble antioxidants are actually absorbed from the intestinal tract, and thus it has been argued that 90 percent of antioxidants are therefore wasted. But this argument has no scientific merit, for the presence of increased amounts of antioxidants in the digestive tract, even if *not absorbed,* markedly reduces the levels of toxins formed during digestion, and thereby may potentially decrease their adverse health effects.

Given this, we believe that moderate supplementation with multiple-micronutrients is necessary for optimal health and disease prevention. The dosage and type of micronutrients needed depend on a person's age and gender, and if one is ill, the type of disease one has, the risk levels of their disease (low-risk or high-risk), and the disease stage (early or advanced).

In this chapter we will provide information as to the specific antioxidant needs of the body, and how they may be met with the supplementation of micronutrients to the diet. We will also amplify our prior discussion of potential risk factors of micronutrient supplementation.

HOW MUCH OF EACH ANTIOXIDANT DO WE ABSORB AND RETAIN?

Vitamin A

Only about 10–20 percent of ingested vitamin A is absorbed from the small intestine. Normal cells characteristically do not take up more than they need in order to function. Liver cells are an exception. Ingested retinyl acetate or the retinyl palmitate form of vitamin A is converted to retinol in the intestine. Retinol is further converted to retinoic acid in the cells; however, most of the body's vitamin A is stored in the liver as retinyl palmitate. Retinol reaches its maximum level in the blood three to six hours after the ingestion of vitamin A and drops to a normal level in about twelve hours.

Beta-carotene

Only about 10 percent of ingested beta-carotene is absorbed from the small intestine. Among vegetarians who do not eat eggs or dairy products, most beta-carotene is converted to vitamin A (retinol), whereas among non-vegetarians (who have sufficient stores of vitamin A) such conversion does not take place. The turnover (rate of degradation and excretion) of beta-carotene in the blood is slow.

Vitamin C

Absorption of vitamin C from the intestine varies from 20 to 80 percent, depending upon the dose. If one consumes 200–500 milligrams of vitamin C, about 50 percent will be absorbed. To reduce the formation of cancer-causing substances in the stomach and intestine, certain amounts of unabsorbed vitamin C may be useful. Once absorbed, vitamin C is rapidly distributed throughout the body. As with vitamin A, normal cells do not take up more vitamin C than they need to function. Vitamin C is rapidly degraded in the body.

Vitamin E

Vitamin E can be taken as alpha-tocopherol, alpha-tocopheryl acetate, or alpha-tocopheryl succinate (vitamin E succinate). If the body stores of alpha-tocopherol are full, a portion of vitamin E succinate is converted to alpha-tocopherol in the intestine before absorption, but the remaining is absorbed without degradation. About 20 percent of ingested vitamin E is absorbed from the intestine and is rapidly distributed in the membranous structures of the cells throughout the body. The maximum levels of vitamin E in the blood appear four to six hours after ingestion. The turnover of vitamin E in the blood is slow.

Coenzyme Q10 and Melatonin

Coenzyme Q10 is made in our body, and its level is relatively constant unless the cells are damaged. The absorption of coenzyme Q10 from the intestinal tract varies, depending upon the preparation.

Ingested melatonin is also absorbed from the small intestine but it is rapidly degraded in the body. This hormone is not recommended as a supplement except occasionally for individuals who have infrequent sleep problems.

Glutathione, N-acetylcysteine, and Alpha-lipoic Acid

Glutathione in solid form is fairly stable at room temperature. Glutathione is a powerful antioxidant inside the cells, but it is very sensitive to oxidative stress, and an increased production of free radicals can diminish it in the cells. Glutathione cannot be taken orally because it is completely degraded in the human intestine. In order to increase the level of glutathione in the body, n-acetylcysteine (NAC), which is degraded only very little in the gut and which raises the level of glutathione in the cells, is recommended.

Alpha-lipoic acid is made in the body. Ingested alpha-lipoic acid is absorbed from the small intestine and is rapidly distributed into various tissues in the body. Its product, dihydrolipoic acid, also acts as an antioxidant. Both substances remove metals from the body. Alpha-lipoic acid also increases the level of glutathione in the body.

Polyphenols

These antioxidants are absorbed from the intestine without significant degradation and are distributed throughout the body. The turnover of phenolic compounds in the blood is slow. These antioxidants are consumed through the diet in large quantities (grams). For this reason, supplements of a few milligrams in pills may not be useful in preventing chronic disease.

WHICH ANTIOXIDANT SUPPLEMENTS SHOULD WE TAKE? HOW MUCH AND HOW OFTEN?

At this time, the correct dosage of antioxidants intended to impart the greatest benefit to human health and a maximum reduction in the incidence of chronic disease is unknown. Nevertheless, 40 percent or more of all Americans take micronutrient supplements, which contain antioxidants, on a regular basis, hoping to improve their health. In addition, many people with chronic diseases take these supplements with or without their doctor's approval. (Many doctors do not recommend micronutrient supplements for optimal health or chronic disease prevention and treatment.)

When one talks with people who are taking micronutrients on the advice of a salesperson at a vitamin store, or because of an article that they read in a health-related magazine or a book, or heard on a television report, it becomes evident that many of them are doing so without reference to scientific rationale. Furthermore, the makers of most multivitamin preparations have not given sufficient attention to the dose, type, and chemical form of antioxidants, or to the appropriate minerals that should be included in their formulation. For example, most commercially sold multivitamin supplements contain the minerals iron, copper, and manganese—or all three.

Iron, copper, and manganese—when combined with vitamin C—generate excessive amounts of free radicals in the body, which can contribute to the development of several chronic diseases, including diabetes. Therefore, the addition of iron, copper, and/or manganese to any multivitamin preparation has no scientific merit in terms of ensuring optimal health or preventing chronic diseases. (In cases where an individual has iron-deficiency anemia, however, a short-term iron supplement with vitamin C is essential to help with iron absorption until the anemia is cured.)

Many commercially sold preparations contain heavy metals such as vanadium and molybdenum, despite the fact that sufficient amounts of them are obtained from a normal diet. The daily consumption of these heavy metals over a long period of time can increase the body's stores of them because the body has no efficient way of eliminating them. The accumulation of excessive amounts of these metals can be toxic to brain cells.

Many commercial supplements also include inositol, methionine, and choline in varying doses (30–60 milligrams). Such doses serve no useful purpose, because the necessary 400 to 1,000 milligrams of them are obtained daily from the diet. Para-aminobenzoic acid (PABA) is present in some multivitamin preparations. PABA has no biological function in the body. In addition, it blocks the anti-bacterial effects of sulfonamides. Therefore, patients taking sulfonamides and a multiple antioxidant containing PABA may experience diminished effectiveness of the antibiotics.

Commercially sold multivitamin preparations often contain n-acetylcysteine (NAC) or alpha-lipoic acid. These agents increase glutathione levels in the cells by different pathways. Therefore, in order to increase the level of glutathione maximally, the addition of both NAC and alpha-lipoic acid in a multivitamin preparation is important.

The addition of both beta-carotene and vitamin A to a multivitamin preparation is also important, because beta-carotene not only acts as a precursor of vitamin A but also has important biological functions that vitamin A does not. Unfortunately, the beneficial effects of beta-carotene have become controversial because of flawed clinical studies that received wide publicity.

Because of this, the addition of beta-carotene to multivitamin preparations has been discouraged, and generally is not approved by the committee responsible for human studies (Institional Review Board or IRB).

Other carotenoids such as lycopene and lutein are also important for health, but they can be obtained from a diet rich in tomatoes (lycopene), spinach (lutein), and paprika (xanthophylls, including lutein) in amounts that are much higher than those found in vitamin supplements. Therefore, the addition of very small amounts of lycopene and lutein to a multivitamin preparation serves no useful purpose for overall health or the prevention of chronic disease. However, having said that, doses of lutein and lycopene that are higher than commonly present in a multivitamin preparation may be needed for the healthy maintenance of vision and for a healthy prostate.

Two forms of vitamin E, alpha-tocopheryl acetate (commonly used in laboratory experiments) and alpha-tocopheryl succinate, should be present in a multivitamin preparation because vitamin E succinate is the most effective form of vitamin E. Laboratory experiments show that alpha-tocopherol (at doses of 20–60 micrograms/milliliter) can increase immune function, but beta-, gamma-, and delta- forms of vitamin E at similar doses can inhibit it. For this reason, supplementation with beta-, gamma-, or delta-tocopherol is not recommended.

Similarly, tocotrienols inhibit cholesterol synthesis. Cholesterol is necessary to maintain the normal functioning of all cells, particularly brain cells. The prolonged inhibition of cholesterol production in healthy persons with normal cholesterol levels may be harmful in young adults; therefore, they cannot be used as supplements for optimal health in this group. In addition, coenzyme Q10 formation occurs in the same pathway as cholesterol. Therefore, a reduction in the level of cholesterol by tocotrienol may also cause a decrease in the level of coenzyme Q10, a necessary substance for the generation of energy in the body.

The optimal form of vitamin C is calcium ascorbate because it is not acidic and does not cause an upset stomach (as ascorbic acid can in some people). The addition of potassium ascorbate or magnesium ascorbate to a multivitamin preparation is unnecessary.

Adequate amounts of B vitamins (two to three times the RDA value) and appropriate minerals such as selenium, zinc, and chromium should be included in a multivitamin preparation. Supplementation with B vitamins is necessary for reducing levels of homocysteine, a risk factor for developing heart disease, and it is essential for maintaining optimal health. Selenium activates the antioxidant enzyme glutathione peroxidase, which makes glutathione.

It is not possible to recommend an appropriate multiple antioxidant supplement that can be useful to everyone, irrespective of age, gender, general health, and disease status. Therefore, a separate multivitamin preparation specific to the health conditions referenced above should be utilized. This issue is discussed in detail in chapter 6.

IF WE EAT A BALANCED DIET, DO WE NEED SUPPLEMENTARY ANTIOXIDANTS FOR OPTIMAL HEALTH AND CHRONIC DISEASE PREVENTION?

The answer to the above-referenced question is yes, although the perception of a balanced diet may differ from one individual to another. Generally, what is meant by a balanced diet is one which is low in fat and high in fiber, and includes plenty of fresh fruits and vegetables. This diet may be sufficient for normal growth and development, but supplementary micronutrients, including dietary and endogenous antioxidants, are important for maintaining optimal health and for disease prevention and treatment. One would have difficulty eating fresh fruits and vegetables daily in the amounts and at the rates that maintain ideal levels of dietary antioxidants in the blood. Furthermore, older individuals have a reduced capacity to make endogenous antioxidants. Given all of these factors, it is important to take an appropriate preparation of micronutrients containing multiple antioxidants, in addition to eating a balanced diet.

It is now known that many foods (even if grown organically) have naturally occurring toxic as well as protective substances. In fact, 90 percent of toxins come from the diet, and only about 1 percent or less are man-made toxins such as pesticides that are sprayed on the agricultural produce we consume. A balanced diet alone cannot get rid of naturally occurring toxins; therefore, diet alone is not sufficient to prevent chronic disease in an optimal manner. While a balanced diet is better than junk food and will protect against vitamin deficiency, the main problem with the concept of such a diet is that it is too general, and its interpretation can vary markedly from one person to another.

For instance, some people believe that a daily intake of one apple, one carrot, one orange, a few fresh vegetables, a little meat, and some carbohydrates constitutes a balanced diet. Other people define a balanced diet differently, with more or less of these same foods. Even if a balanced diet is defined and standardized, the same diet cannot be applied to all regions of the world because dietary and environmental toxin levels vary markedly from one region to another.

It is important to realize that some toxic agents such as pesticides are synthetic, whereas most, such as mutagens and carcinogens, are found in nature. The risk of chronic illness, including diabetes, may depend in part upon the relative consumption of protective versus toxic substances. If the daily intake of protective substances is higher than that of toxic agents, the risk of chronic disease may be lower. Since we know very little about the relative levels of toxic and protective substances in any diet, we cannot know whether we are consuming higher levels of protective substances compared with toxic ones. To ensure a higher intake of protective agents, it is important to take daily a preparation of micronutrients containing dietary and endogenous antioxidants.

A CLOSER LOOK AT THE TOXICITY OF MICRONUTRIENTS

Vitamin A

Liver toxicity and skin reactions have been noted after the oral ingestion of 50,000 IU per day of vitamin A for a year or more. Some of these changes are reversible when the vitamin is discontinued. Liver toxicity can be irreversible. Up to 5,000 IU of vitamin A, taken orally and divided into two doses (morning and evening) per day, is unlikely to produce major toxic effects in a normal adult. Higher doses of vitamin A have been associated with an increased risk of bone fracture in older individuals. As mentioned in the last chapter, the ingestion of vitamin A at doses of 10,000 IU per day can increase the risk of birth defects in pregnant women. Because of these toxicities, the Recommended Dietary Allowance (RDA) of vitamin A for adults has been reduced from 5,000

IU to 3,000 IU per day. Pregnant women should avoid taking more than 3,000 IU of vitamin A daily. Retinoic acid and other derivatives of vitamin A should not be consumed orally for general health maintenance because of the toxic effects of these compounds at low doses.

Beta-carotene

The toxicity of beta-carotene has become a controversial issue. A few studies have suggested that taking synthetic beta-carotene at a daily dose of 25 milligrams alone can increase the risk of cancer and some forms of heart disease among groups of people who are at higher-than-average risk of developing heart disease and diabetes (such as men who are heavy tobacco smokers and those who are obese). This was not an unexpected result because the bodies of heavy tobacco smokers have a highly oxidative environment in which beta-carotene is readily oxidized and can act as a pro-oxidant rather than as an antioxidant. There are no studies that show that if beta-carotene is present in a multiple antioxidant preparation it will increase the risk of developing diabetes or heart disease among high-risk populations.

There is no known toxicity of beta-carotene in amounts up to 15 milligrams/day in a multivitamin preparation in normal persons or high-risk populations. As discussed earlier, bronzing of the skin may appear after oral ingestion of beta-carotene at 100 milligrams/day or more over a few months. Deposits of beta-carotene pigment are found in the eye after long-term consumption of high doses of beta-carotene. Excessive deposits of this pigment can harm the eye. These changes are reversible upon a discontinuation of the supplement.

The other carotenoids such as lutein and lycopene are nontoxic at oral doses of up to 25 milligrams per day.

Vitamin C

In most healthy people, doses of vitamin C up to 10 grams per day taken orally will not produce any toxic effects. Intravenous infusions of vitamin C at doses of 50 grams or more have produced no significant toxic effects on blood profiles of cancer patients. And although we have previously cited how harmful it is to have high levels of certain minerals in the body, this information bears repeating again. Some diseases involving iron metabolism (such as hemochromatosis, wherein the body has very high levels of iron), or copper metabolism (for example, Wilson's disease in which the body has excessive amounts of copper), or exposure to high levels of manganese (symptoms akin to those found with Parkinson's disease), the excessive consumption of vitamin C may be harmful because vitamin C in combination with iron, copper, and/or manganese, in the presence of oxygen, generates excessive amounts of free radicals.

As regards kidney stones and gout, there is no scientific evidence to show that vitamin C supplementation in a multivitamin preparation at high doses raises the risk of these two conditions in most normal people. As mentioned previously, increased urinary excretion of oxalic acid in people taking high doses of vitamin C has been interpreted to mean that this vitamin may increase the risk of kidney stones, since the increased excretion of oxalic acid is also found in many patients with kidney stones. These could be the result of independent biochemical reactions, however, and the two events may not necessarily be linked. (There were no documented cases of an elevated incidence of kidney stones among any study group taking high doses of vitamin C that had been included in a multiple-micronutrient preparation.)

I recommend that up to 2 grams/day of vitamin C be added to a multiple-micronutrient preparation, which should be taken orally twice a day. This dose of vitamin C is safe in most healthy adults.

Vitamin E

High doses of vitamin E (2,000 IU daily) can, as previously discussed, cause a blood-clotting defect, which is reversible after the administration of vitamin K.

According to many studies, up to 400 IU of vitamin E present in a multivitamin preparation per day is safe in most healthy adults.

However, the same dose of vitamin E alone, if taken orally, may increase the risk of some forms of heart disease in high-risk populations such as heavy tobacco smokers or individuals with a previous history of heart disease. This is due to the fact that the bodies of these high-risk individuals are highly oxidative (vitamin E is more apt to be oxidized and act as a pro-oxidant rather than as an antioxidant). This is similar to what happens with relatively the same group as regards beta-carotene, discussed above.

Coenzyme Q10

Oral doses of up to 300 milligrams of coenzyme Q10 have been given to patients with breast cancer, and up to 1,200 milligrams to patients with Parkinson's disease without significant apparent toxicity. High doses of coenzyme Q10 have also been used in the treatment of advanced heart disease without adverse effects. Doses of up to 200 milligrams in a multivitamin preparation, taken orally every day, are considered safe for most adults.

Glutathione, N-acetylcysteine (NAC), and Alpha-lipoic Acid

Glutathione is considered non-toxic at doses commonly used; however, it cannot be absorbed when ingested orally because it is totally degraded in the intestinal tract.

N-acetylcysteine is commonly used to increase levels of glutathione in the body. Doses of up to 300–400 milligrams in a multivitamin preparation are considered safe. High doses of NAC can bind with heavy metals such as lead, and mercury and remove them from the body, but if such doses are ingested on a regular basis they can increase the excretion of valuable minerals such as zinc, which can be harmful.

Similarly to NAC, alpha-lipoic acid is also considered a metal chelator (capable of removing metal from the body). For this reason, long-term consumption at high doses (300 milligrams or more) may induce the deficiency of some important metals necessary to the body's overall health and optimal functioning.

Polyphenols

Although polyphenols have no known toxicity at doses used in several laboratory and human studies, the adverse health effects of high doses of these compounds have not been evaluated in humans.

Selenium and Zinc

An antioxidant enzyme, glutathione peroxidase, requires selenium in order to exert its antioxidant action. Selenium in combination with vitamin E is more effective than either micronutrient taken alone. Certain metals such as lead, cadmium, arsenic, mercury, and silver block the action of selenium.

Commercial preparations of selenium include inorganic selenium (sodium selenite) and various forms of organic selenium. Some studies have reported that sodium selenite is not absorbed adequately, whereas organic selenium, including yeast-selenium and seleno-L-methionine, is absorbed very well. For this reason, seleno-L-methionine is the form of selenium that is most commonly used in a multivitamin preparation.

The optimal doses of selenium in terms of its health benefits are unknown. In the United States, the average dietary intake of selenium is about 125–150 micrograms per day. The RDA value of selenium for adults is 55–70 micrograms per day. If an average person consumes 125–150 micrograms of selenium each day, a supplement of 100 micrograms of selenium in a multivitamin preparation is safe. High doses of selenium (400 micrograms or more), if ingested every day for a long period of time, may induce dry skin and cataract formation in some individuals.

It is a common belief that high doses of zinc are important for maintaining good health, but this may not be true. Several laboratory experiments have shown that high doses of zinc block the action of selenium. Furthermore, high doses of zinc can damage mitochondrial function, thereby increasing the production of free radicals. Thus, doses higher than 15–25 milligrams of zinc in a multivitamin preparation should be avoided.

ADVERSE HEALTH EVENTS ASSOCIATED WITH MICRONUTRIENT SUPPLEMENTATION

Since the mandatory reporting of adverse health events in association with the consumption of dietary supplements went into effect in 2007, the Government Accountability Office (GAO) found a threefold increase in the number of all adverse health events compared with the previous year. The FDA estimates the total number of adverse health events that are related to the consumption of the dietary supplements to be over 50,000 per year. These adverse health events occurred primarily as a result of the consumption of certain herbs such as Ephedra, which is considered a dietary supplement. Other types of dietary supplements, such as vitamins A, C, E, carotenoids, glutathione, R-alpha-lipoic acid, coenzyme Q10, and L-carnitine, have not produced any adverse health events for decades. However, the reported adverse health effects of certain herbs were perceived by most consumers to include the above-referenced antioxidants. I strongly believe that reporting of any adverse effects of certain herbs should be specific to those herbs and not to other dietary supplements such as antioxidants.

Similarly, the reporting of adverse effects obtained from the use of a single antioxidant such as beta-carotene, in populations at high risk to develop cancer or heart disease, should not conclude that taking beta-carotene in a multiple antioxidant preparation would produce results similar to that produced by beta-carotene alone. In addition, the results obtained from populations at high risk to develop cancer, heart disease, or diabetes should not be extrapolated to be the same as for healthy adults. Unfortunately, most reports that are published state that antioxidants can increase the risk of cancer as well as heart disease in populations that are at high risk for developing chronic diseases.

This erroneous reporting of scientific observations (based on the use of a single antioxidant) creates uncertainty and anxiety in the minds of those who are taking or who may want to take dietary supplements. This is a great disservice to those who are seeking to optimize their health and well-being through micronutrient supplementation.

VITAMIN CONSUMPTION AND ITS COST

In 2009, it was estimated that more than 50 percent of adults in the United States consume some form of dietary supplements (National Health Interview Survey 2009). In 2007, the sales of dietary supplements reached 23.7 billion dollars. And despite media reports of inconsistent and occasionally negative results obtained from some flawed clinical studies in which a single antioxidant was used for populations at a high risk of developing heart disease, the number of consumers of dietary supplements has not declined.

The number of dietary supplements in the marketplace rose from about 4,000 in 1995 to about 75,000 in 2008. In addition, innumerable food products such as fortified cereals and energy drinks, which contain a variety of dietary supplements, are now widely available to consumers.

CONCLUDING REMARKS

In this chapter we have taken a closer look at some different aspects of micronutrients in order to determine if our body's needs for them are being met. Absorption is a key factor in this regard. It is also imperative to understand what a proper dosing schedule should look like, as well as determine which substances may be toxic to us in ways previously overlooked. And although we may believe that we receive adequate micronutrient supplementation from our diet, we have examined how fallacious this reasoning may be.

We have also learned that while most antioxidants at certain doses are considered safe, some antioxidants such as vitamin A, beta-carotene, and vitamin E at high doses can be harmful after long-term daily consumption. It is also important to understand how the media frequently distorts the truth about micronutrient supplementation.

In the next chapter we will look more closely at the relationship of micronutrients to the prevention of diabetes, most specifically via clinical studies that have been done, which have studied the effects of same.

5 The Search for Prevention Part 1

The Laboratory and Epidemiologic Studies

In taking a closer look at the potentially preventive and therapeutic effects of supplements in the prevention and treatment of diabetes, in this chapter we will discuss studies that have been done on this topic. The laboratory experiments have been done on animals. Human studies have been performed utilizing epidemiologic studies (survey-types of studies) and intervention studies. Almost all of these studies used only one or a few supplementary agents as variables. As will become clear later in the book, this author maintains that these studies are limited because of this, and advocates instead for the need for clinical studies utilizing a multiple-micronutrient formula. In chapter 6, we will go on to look at the results of clinical intervention studies, to determine the effectiveness of micronutrients in combating diabetes.

ANIMAL STUDIES WITH MICRONUTRIENTS

Animal studies are considered essential by most investigators prior to testing the value of micronutrients for the prevention or improved treatment of diabetes in humans. However, some scientists believe that extensive use of animals in micronutrient research is not warranted, and that most study results—such as beneficial or toxic effects—can be obtained from studying normal human cell cultures. Although the mechanisms for the development of diabetes, and risk factors that can initiate and promote this development, *can* be studied in cell-culture models, the clinical markers of diabetes—hyperglycemia, insulin release, insulin sensitivity, and diabetes-related complications (damage to the eyes, kidneys, and nervous system)—cannot. Instead, these can easily be studied in chemically induced diabetes in animals. (The most commonly used chemicals for inducing type 1 diabetes or type 2 diabetes are streptozotocin and alloxan.)

Animal studies are relatively easy and inexpensive compared to human studies. In addition, the results of the animal models of diabetes can be obtained within a few months rather than a few years. It should be always remembered, however, that animal studies provide only a *guide* with respect to the effectiveness of supplements in reducing the risk of diabetes in humans. The effective dose, dose-schedule, safety, and period of observation used in animal experiments cannot be used in the experimental design of human studies.

This is due to the fact that the extent of effectiveness, absorption, metabolism (turnover), excretion, and toxicity of antioxidants and vitamins in animals are different than those for humans. In addition, most mammals, except guinea pigs, make their own vitamin C, whereas humans do not; humans rely on their diet for vitamin C. This is significant because the presence of vitamin C in most animals can influence the effectiveness of antioxidant supplementation in reducing the risk of diabetes.

Some animal studies detailing the effects of antioxidants, omega-3 fatty acids, and aspirin are described next.

Vitamin A

It has been suggested that a decreased production of nerve growth factor (NGF) may contribute to diabetic neuropathy (damage to the nerves); however, the administration of exogenous NGF produced only a modest benefit. Retinoic acid (RA), a metabolite of retinol (vitamin A), induced expression of NGF and its receptor (Hernandez-Pedro et al. 2008). Therefore, it is thought that the administration of retinoic acid may be useful in improving some of the symptoms of diabetes-related damage to nerve cells (neuropathy).

Indeed, treatment of streptozotocin-induced diabetic mice with RA increased levels of NGF in serum and in nerve cells, and induced nerve regeneration (Hernandez-Pedro et al. 2008); however, the levels of plasma glucose did not change, and there was no difference in the pain threshold among treated and untreated groups of diabetic animals.

An elevated level of serum retinol-binding protein-4 (RBP-4) secreted from adipose tissue (fat) plays an important role in the development of insulin resistance. Therefore, lowering the level of RBP-4 may increase the sensitivity of cells to insulin for glucose uptake. Administration of all-retinoic acid reduced body weight, serum glucose, retinol, and RBP-4, and also improved insulin sensitivity in diabetic mice (Manolescu et al. 2010). Thus, vitamin A supplementation alone was not effective in reducing diabetes-related retinopathy, but was effective in improving insulin sensitivity.

Type 1 diabetes is characterized by inflammation, as evidenced by the infiltration of activated T-lymphocytes and monocytes into the islet cells of the pancreas, resulting in a loss of beta-cells (cells that produce insulin). Supplementation with vitamin A (retinyl acetate), or polyphenols through diet caused a marked reduction in the inflammatory molecule TNF-alpha (tumor necrosis factor–alpha) and a loss of beta-cells in diabetic mice (Zunino et al. 2007).

Retinoic acid suppresses adipogenesis (the formation of fat), and this property of retinoic acid may be responsible for preventing diet-induced obesity (Berry et al. 2012). Vitamin A supplementation in this study appears to be useful in preventing the loss of beta-cells from the pancreas and thus could be useful in preventing the development of type 1 diabetes.

The studies discussed above suggest that vitamin A supplementation alone may help in reducing some diabetes-related complications, but by itself it is not optimal for reducing the risk of developing diabetes or preventing all diabetes-related complications.

Vitamin C

Treatment of streptozotocin-induced diabetic rats with vitamin C suppressed leukocyte adhesion and endothelial dysfunction (defects in the dilation of blood vessels), and improved blood flow in the microvessels (the tiny blood vessels that feed blood to the eyes) of the iris of the eyes (Jariyapongskul et al. 2007).

Vitamin C treatment in diabetic rats also prevented diabetic-induced endothelial dysfunction (abnormal blood-vessel function) (Sridulyakul et al. 2006). Abnormal blood-vessel function can increase the risk of diabetes-related complications including heart disease.

These studies suggest that vitamin C supplementation may be of some value in preventing diabetes-related retinopathy (damage to the eyes).

Increased oxidative stress also plays an important role in causing diabetes-related kidney damage (nephropathy). This is shown by the fact that supplementation with vitamin C in the diabetic rat model reduced damage to the kidneys without changing the level of plasma glucose (Lee et al. 2007). This suggested that vitamin C reduced oxidative stress to the kidneys, although it had no role in regulating plasma glucose levels.

Administration of vitamin C (200 milligrams/kilogram of body weight) orally into streptozotocin-induced diabetic rats improved gastric secretion and protected against the development of ulcers in the intestine (Owu et al. 2012).

In streptozotocin-induced type 1 diabetic rats, the function of T-lymphocytes is damaged. Treatment of diabetic animals with vitamin C (60 milligrams/kilogram of body weight) restored the normal function of T-lymphocytes (Badr et al. 2012). Abnormal functioning of T-lymphocytes may increase the risk of autoimmunity that plays an important role in the loss of beta-cells from the pancreas in type 1 diabetes.

The studies discussed above suggest that vitamin C supplementation alone may help in reducing some diabetes-related complications, but by itself is not optimal for reducing the risk of developing diabetes or preventing all diabetes-related complications.

Vitamin D

In a rat model of diabetes, the administration of 1alpha,25-dihydroxyvitamin D_3 (1alpha, 25(OH) 2-VD_3: vitamin D_3) increased plasma insulin levels, normalized the hepatic glycogen concentration, and maintained normal plasma glucose levels. In addition, treatment with vitamin D_3 enhanced the activities of the antioxidant enzymes superoxide dismutase (SOD), catalase, and glutathione peroxidase in diabetic rats compared to diabetic rats that did not receive vitamin D_3. It also reduced lipid peroxidation and damage to the liver and kidneys (Hamden et al. 2009).

Vitamin D deficiency may be associated with both type 1 and type 2 diabetes, and it impairs biosynthesis and the release of insulin in animals and humans with type 2 diabetes. In non-obese diabetic mice, supplementation with vitamin D_3 or its analogs delayed the onset of diabetes (Mathieu et al. 2005; Palomer et al. 2008).

These studies suggest that the administration of vitamin D alone may have a role in reducing the risk of developing type 2 diabetes and may improve some symptoms of diabetes in animal models.

Vitamin E

It has been reported that an oral administration of vitamin E reduced kidney malondialdehyde (MDA: a marker of oxidative stress), in both diabetic and control rats (Ulusu et al. 2003). Haptoglobin (Hp) is an antioxidant protein that protects against oxidative damage caused by extracorpuscular hemoglobin (free hemoglobin in plasma). There are two alleles at the Hp locus: 1 and 2. The Hp-1 is a superior antioxidant compared to Hp-2. The haptoglobin (Hp) 2-2 genotype is associated with an increased risk of diabetes. This genotype is also associated with an increased risk of diabetic nephropathy (kidney disease) and appears to be associated with a more rapid progression to end-stage renal disease.

Using transgenic mice, it was demonstrated that vitamin E supplementation provided significant protection against the development of diabetic kidney disease in mice with the Hp2-2 genotype, but not in mice with the Hp1-1 genotype (Nakhoul et al. 2009). This study supports the idea that the HP2-2 gene plays a role in the development of diabetes-related kidney disease. This study also reveals that vitamin E interacts with the Hp2-2 gene in order to protect the kidney from the development of kidney disease in mice.

It has been reported that administration of tocotrienol, a form of vitamin E (25 milligrams, 50 milligrams, and 100 milligrams/kilogram of body weight), was effective in protecting against diabetes-related kidney disease in streptozotocin-induced diabetic rats. Tocotrienol (100 milligrams/kilogram of body weight) was more effective than the same dose of alpha-tocopherol (Kuhad and Chopra 2009).

In a rat model of type 1 diabetes induced by streptozotocin, supplementation with vitamin E (2,000 IU/kilogram of body weight) reduced markers of oxidative stress in the heart, damage to heart muscle, and the incidence of heart failure (Hamblin et al. 2007).

The studies discussed above suggest that vitamin E supplementation alone may help in reducing some of the diabetes-related complications; however, it is not optimal for reducing the risk of developing diabetes or preventing all diabetes-related complications.

A Combination of Vitamins C and E

Supplementation with vitamin C and vitamin E reduced damage to the kidneys and the eyes in aged streptozotocin-induced diabetic rats (Ozkaya et al. 2011).

Learning and memory loss occur in patients with diabetes. It was demonstrated that the administration of vitamin C (50 milligrams/

kilogram of body weight) and vitamin E (100 milligrams/kilogram of body weight) improved learning ability and memory in normal rats and reversed memory loss in diabetic rats (Hasanein and Shahidi 2010).

These studies suggest that supplementation with a combination of vitamin E and vitamin C reduced some diabetes-related complications; however, the two antioxidants taken together are not optimal for reducing the risk of developing diabetes or preventing all diabetes-related complications.

Alpha-lipoic Acid

The enzyme lipoic acid synthase is involved in the formation of new alpha-lipoic acid. In the animal model of diabetes type 2, the expression of the gene that codes for this enzyme is significantly reduced. Reduced levels of alpha-lipoic acid synthase aggravated the pro-inflammatory responses, whereas over-expression of this gene prevented inflammatory responses in diabetic animals (Padmalayam et al. 2009).

It has been reported that supplementation with alpha-lipoic acid reduced neural tube defects, cardiovascular malformations, and skeletal muscle malformations in the offspring of diabetic mice at term delivery (Sugimura et al. 2009).

Supplementation with alpha-lipoic acid delayed the development and progression of diabetes-related cataracts in streptozotocin-induced diabetic rats (Kojima et al. 2007).

It has been reported that the combination of alpha-lipoic acid and pyridoxamine (a form of vitamin B_6 found in food) produced better results in insulin-mediated glucose transport in the soleus muscles of obese Zucker rats with insulin resistance, compared to those produced by alpha-lipoic acid alone (Muellenbach et al. 2008). This study suggests that the addition of B vitamins is important for improving the beneficial effects of alpha-lipoic acid.

In a diabetic rat model, supplementation with alpha-lipoic acid reduced proteinuria (proteins secreted in the urine due to damage to the kidneys), which contributes to diabetic nephropathy (Lee et al.

2009). Thus, supplementation with alpha-lipoic acid may help prevent the development of kidney disease in diabetic animals.

From all of these animal studies, it appears that supplementation with alpha-lipoic acid may prevent some diabetes-related complications, such as damage to the eyes, nerve cells, and the kidneys.

Coenzyme Q10

Diabetes and obesity can be induced by consumption of excessive dietary fat that increases the levels of markers of oxidative stress and inflammation. It has been reported that supplementation with coenzyme Q10 reduced expressions of inflammatory genes without changing the levels of lipid peroxides in the liver of mice that were fed a high-fat diet, compared to control mice receiving a high-fat diet but no coenzyme Q10 (Sohet et al. 2009). This study suggests that coenzyme Q10 supplementation reduced inflammation without affecting oxidative stress in mice that were fed a high-fat diet.

The treatment of human umbilical-vein epithelial cells in culture with coenzyme Q10 prevented hyperglycemia-induced increased oxidative stress and inflammation (Tsuneki et al. 2007). This suggests that coenzyme Q10 can protect against hyperglycemia-induced endothelial dysfunction, which increases the progression of cardiovascular disease in diabetes.

Neuropathy, a disorder of nerve conduction, is associated with type 2 diabetes. Supplementation with coenzyme Q10 improved nerve conduction in diabetic rats (Ayaz et al. 2008).

These studies suggest that supplementation with coenzyme Q10 treatment can help improve nerve conduction and the function of blood vessels in patients with type 2 diabetes.

L-carnitine

Obesity can contribute to glucose intolerance. It has been reported that supplementation with L-carnitine improved insulin-stimulated glucose uptake and the utilization of glucose in genetically induced diabetic mice and wild-type mice (normal mice without a genetic alteration) that were fed a high-fat diet (Power et al. 2007).

Diabetes is known to cause impaired nerve conduction. Using streptozotocin-induced diabetic rats, it has been demonstrated that supplementation with a high dose of acetyl-L-carnitine improved nerve conduction; however, a lower dose of acetyl-L-carnitine was less effective (Soneru et al. 1997).

Glycation refers to a process in which glucose attaches to proteins or fats without the help of an enzyme. Increased levels of advanced glycation end-products (AGE) are present in patients with diabetes. A high-fructose diet caused the development of hyperglycemia and glycation of hemoglobin; however, supplementation with L-carnitine significantly reduced glycation of hemoglobin. The efficacy of L-carnitine in reducing glycation was compared with a well-known anti-glycation agent, aminoguanidine. The results showed that L-carnitine was more effective than aminoguanidine in inhibiting glycation in vitro (cells in petri dishes) (Rajasekar and Anuradha 2007).

Streptozotocin-induced diabetes in rats is associated with L-carnitine deficiency and can cause abnormal heart function. An oral supplementation of L-carnitine normalized serum L-carnitine and restored heart function to a normal level (Malone et al. 2006).

Excessive administration of insulin can cause hypoglycemia (a less than normal plasma level of glucose) that can induce mitochondrial swelling, eventually causing the death of neurons in the brain. The administration of L-carnitine prevented neuronal damage to the brain in insulin-induced hypoglycemic rats by improving mitochondrial function (Hino et al. 2005).

These studies suggest that supplementation with L-carnitine may reduce some symptoms of diabetes and some diabetes-related complications.

N-acetylcysteine (NAC)

In a rat model of type 1 diabetes, administration of NAC reduced the levels of hyperglycemia-induced oxidative stress (Kamboj et al. 2009).

Increased markers of oxidative stress and inflammation appear to be associated with diabetic retinopathy (damage to the eyes). Supplementation with NAC reduced the levels of these markers in streptozotocin-induced diabetic rats (Tsai et al. 2009), and thus may help reduce the risk of retinopathy.

Hyperglycemia-induced increased oxidative stress is also involved in the development of cardiomyopathy (damage to the heart's muscle cells) associated with diabetes. Supplementation with NAC reduced markers of oxidative stress and prevented hyperglycemia-induced cardiomyocyte damage in cultured neonatal cardiomyocytes (Xia et al. 2007).

Hyperglycemia-induced oxidative stress is associated with diabetic encephalopathy (damage to the brain), which impairs cognitive function. Supplementation with NAC via drinking water significantly reduced cognitive deficits and oxidative stress in streptozotocin-induced diabetic rats (Kamboj et al. 2008).

Diabetes in pregnant women increases the risk for congenital heart disease in offspring. NAC-treatment reduced diabetes-related dysfunction of the heart by restoring heart Mn-SOD (manganese-dependent superoxide dismutase) activity (Xia et al. 2006).

These studies suggest that NAC supplementation was of some value in reducing the risk of some complications related to diabetes.

Multiple Antioxidants

A mixture of vitamin C, vitamin E, and selenium protected the lens of the eyes of streptozotocin-induced diabetic rats against oxidative damage by reducing markers of oxidative damage and improving the antioxidant defense system (Naziroglu et al. 1999).

Oral administration of vitamin C (250 milligrams/kilogram of body weight), vitamin E (250 milligrams/kilogram of body weight), and selenium (0.2 milligrams/kilogram of body weight) into streptozotocin-induced diabetic rats decreased lipid peroxidation, improved glutathione levels in the skin, and prevented damage to the skin (Sokmen et al. 2012).

Treatment of diabetic rats with beta-carotene, pycnogenol, and alpha-lipoic acid alone or in combination normalized lipid peroxidation in the liver, kidneys, and heart. Glutathione is the most important antioxidant inside of the cells to protect against oxidative damage and this mixture of antioxidants elevated glutathione levels and glutathione peroxidase activity in the heart (Berryman et al. 2004).

In streptozotocin-induced diabetic rats, supplementation with curcumin and vitamin C together was more effective in reducing blood glucose, glycosylated hemoglobin (HbA1c), lipid abnormalities, leukocyte adhesion, and MDA (melondialdehyde) than the individual agents working alone (Patumraj et al. 2006).

It has also been reported that a combination of vitamin E and magnesium was more effective in improving plasma lipid abnormalities and blood viscosity in diabetic rats than the individual agents working alone (Dou et al. 2009).

Additionally, it has been demonstrated that dietary supplementation with 0.5 percent vitamin C, 0.5 percent vitamin E, and 2.5 percent n-acetylcysteine improved blood glucose and wound-healing rates in alloxan monohydrate-induced diabetic mice (Park et al. 2011).

None of the studies above have utilized a full complement of dietary and endogenous antioxidants. Therefore, they have not produced an optimal benefit in reducing the risk of developing diabetes or diabetes-related complications.

Omega-3 Fatty Acids

Omega-3 polyunsaturated fatty acids (n-3-PUFA, also called omega-3 fatty acids) from seafood sources contain eicosapentaenoic acid (EPA) and docosahexaenoic acid (DHA). Omega-3 fatty acids from plant sources contain alpha-linolenic acid (ALA). Omega-3 fatty acids from both seafood and plant sources have been used to investigate the role of omega-3 fatty acids in reducing both the risk of diabetes and diabetes-related complications in animal and human studies.

A few arbitrarily selected animal studies are summarized as follows:

High dietary intake of omega-3 fatty acids reduced diabetes-related kidney disease in diabetic models of rodents (Garman et al. 2009).

Supplementation with omega-3 fatty acids in diabetic animals reduced the levels of MDA (a marker of oxidative stress), and increased activities of antioxidant enzymes SOD (superoxide dismutase) and catalase, and decreased the death of brain neurons (Cosar et al. 2008).

Long-term consumption of a diet rich in omega-3 fatty acids improved blood lipids and vascular function in an animal model of insulin resistance and type 2 diabetes; however, only dietary monosaturated fatty acids and alpha linolenic acid enhanced insulin sensitivity and glycemic responses (Mustad et al. 2006).

Increased inflammation in white adipose tissue (fat) appears to be associated with obesity and type 2 diabetes. In obese mice with diabetes, treatment with omega-3 fatty acids prevented the inflammation of white adipose tissue, which was induced by a high-fat diet (Todoric et al. 2006).

Dietary intake of low-dose omega-3 fatty acids attenuated leukocyte adhesion and leukocyte infiltration into tissues of diabetic mice that were suffering complications from sepsis (Chiu et al. 2007). Supplementation with omega-3 fatty acids in pregnant female diabetic rats improved lipid profiles and antioxidant enzyme activities and the levels of antioxidants (vitamins A, C, and E) in mothers as well as in their offspring (Yessoufou et al. 2006).

Animal studies revealed that supplementation with omega-3 fatty acids may reduce the risk of developing some diabetes-related complications such as damage to the kidneys. Omega-3 fatty acids also serve to reduce oxidative stress and inflammation. This suggests that omega-3 fatty acids from both fish and plant sources should be utilized in order to produce an optimal beneficial effect in the treatment of diabetes.

Aspirin

There are substantial data to show that supplementation with aspirin helped prevent the development of type 2 diabetes by reducing insulin resistance in streptozotocin-treated rats. It also protected the pancreas against streptozotocin-induced damage and maintained near normal levels of glucose in diabetic rats (Martha et al. 2009).

Aspirin treatment protected lacrimal glands (responsible for the production of tears) against damage produced by increased oxidative stress and inflammation in streptozotocin-induced diabetic rats (Jorge et al. 2009).

Pre-treatment with aspirin decreased brain ischemia (a reduced oxygen supply) in diabetic rats, and decreased neurological deficits. It also reduced platelet aggregation. However, aspirin treatment did not alter the levels of glucose and insulin in diabetic rats (Wang et al. 2009).

In diet-induced obese rats, the levels of markers of oxidative damage are increased. Aspirin treatment not only reduced the levels of markers of oxidative damage, but also improved insulin sensitivity in obese rats (Carvalho-Filho et al. 2009).

These studies suggest that treatment with aspirin may be useful in reducing markers of oxidative damage and improving insulin sensitivity in diabetic animals.

THE DESIGN OF HUMAN EPIDEMIOLOGIC STUDIES

Human studies are very expensive and time-consuming, but they are essential to demonstrate the potential of vitamins and antioxidants in reducing the risk of developing diabetes. Human studies are performed in two different ways. One is to perform an epidemiologic study (survey-type of study) and the other is to perform an intervention study in which one group of patients receives oral supplementation of vitamins and the other group receives placebo pills in a similar manner.

Epidemiologic studies are time- and labor-intensive, but less expensive and easier to perform than intervention studies. However, these survey-types of studies can only establish an *association* between an intake of vitamins and antioxidants from the diet and the risk of developing diabetes. Intervention studies, on the other hand, provide *conclusive proof* regarding the effectiveness of vitamins and antioxidants in reducing the risk of developing diabetes.

There are two types of epidemiologic studies. One is called a *retrospective case-control* study, and the other is called a *prospective case-control* study. A *retrospective case-control study* involves an analysis of an individual's past history of dietary intake. Thus, patients are provided with a set of questions about their past history (last week, last month, last year, etc.) of dietary patterns and intake of vitamin supplements, their gender, age, weight, and lifestyle (smoking, stress, physical activity, etc.). From the answers obtained regarding diet and vitamin supplement intake, the levels of intake of vitamins and antioxidants are determined through the use of appropriate nutritional computer software.

These patients are divided into at least two major groups: one group has the highest intake of antioxidants from diet or supplements; the other group has the lowest levels of antioxidant intake. The risk of developing diabetes is then compared between the two groups. (Age, gender, and other confounding factors such as smoking and lifestyle-related variables are generally matched between the two groups.) From this comparison, an association between the levels of intake of vitamins from diet or supplements and diabetes is established.

The association could be that an intake of vitamins from diet or from supplements reduced the risk of developing diabetes or that it had no effect or that it had harmful effects. Generally, in epidemiologic studies, the dietary patterns and vitamin supplements—with respect to the types, doses, dose-schedule, or the number of vitamins—differ markedly from one individual to another. Therefore, it is difficult to make an association between an increased intake of antioxidants from diet or supplements and a reduced risk of developing diabetes.

A *prospective case-control* study involves an analysis of dietary intake from diet records in which participants write down every meal's contents and amount every day for the entire study period. A set of questions regarding diet and vitamin supplements, gender, age, weight, and lifestyle (smoking, stress, physical activity, etc.) is provided to the patient in order to establish baseline information before the start of the experiment. The participating individuals are given a record book with the above-referenced set of questions and asked to write down daily dietary contents, and amounts of vitamin supplements, if any.

At the end of the testing period (generally five to ten years), the intake vitamins from the dietary records of participating individuals is estimated, using appropriate nutritional computer software. The risk of diabetes between those who had a higher intake of vitamins and those who had a lower intake of vitamins is compared. The association could be that a higher intake of vitamins reduced the development of diabetes or had no effect or had harmful effects.

Generally, in this latter type of epidemiologic study, the dietary patterns and vitamin supplements—with respect to the types, doses, dose-schedule, and the number of vitamins—differ markedly from one individual to another. Therefore it is difficult to make an association between an increased intake of antioxidants from diet or vitamin supplements and a reduced risk of developing diabetes. However, this type of survey is more useful than a retrospective case-control study because the information about a person's diet, supplements, and lifestyle is obtained from a record book written daily during the period of experiment, rather than based on a person's past memory.

In any case, the results (positive or negative) of epidemiologic studies alone cannot be used to develop a public policy for recommending vitamin supplements for reducing the risk of diabetes.

EPIDEMIOLOGIC STUDIES
WITH MICRONUTRIENTS

A few examples of epidemiologic studies with antioxidants, omega-3 fatty acids, and aspirin are described here.

Vitamin A

In a study involving twenty-seven pregnant women with gestational diabetes or type 1 diabetes, and twenty-seven healthy, pregnant women, the levels of MDA (malondialdehyde), vitamin A, vitamin E, and the activities of glutathione peroxidase (GPX), and superoxide dismutase (SOD) were determined. The results showed that the pregnant women with gestational diabetes or type 1 diabetes had higher levels of MDA and lower levels of vitamin A and vitamin E. In addition, the activity of the enzyme glutathione peroxidase (GPX), responsible for making glutathione, was lower in the women who had gestational diabetes and type 1 diabetes, whereas the activity of SOD was lower only in women with type 1 diabetes (Peuchant et al. 2004).

In about 42 percent of patients with type 2 diabetes, an increased level of vitamin A was found in their urine (Gavrilov et al. 2012). This study suggests that an elevated urinary vitamin A level may be a sign of damage to the kidneys, given that the increased excretion of vitamin A into the urine may be a sign of heightened oxidative stress in the body.

In a clinical study involving twenty-three pregnant women with type 1 diabetes who subsequently developed preeclampsia (gestational hypertension), and twenty-seven pregnant women with type 1 diabetes who did not develop preeclampsia, the levels of carotenoids (alpha- and beta-carotene, lycopene, and lutein), vitamin A, vitamin E, and vitamin D were measured. The results showed that in women with type 1 diabetes, lower levels of serum alpha- and beta-carotene, as well as vitamin D, were associated with the subsequent development of preeclampsia (Azar et al. 2011).

The levels of serum retinol binding proteins -4 (RBP-4) increased in pregnancy, independent of age and body mass index (BMI); however, the levels were further elevated in pregnant women with gestational diabetes compared to non-diabetic pregnant women (Su et al. 2010).

In another study, the level of RBP-4 was not associated with pregnant women with or without gestational diabetes (Tepper et al. 2010). The reasons for this conflicting result are unknown. However, one study suggested that it is the higher ratio of RBP-4 relative to retinol (vitamin A) that is an important indicator of type 2 diabetes (Erikstrup et al. 2009).

In a Swedish clinical study (Uppsala Longitudinal Study of Adult Men) involving 846 non-diabetic fifty-year-old men, the serum concentration of beta-carotene was correlated with insulin resistance and type 2 diabetes (Arnlov et al. 2009). The results showed that during twenty-seven years of follow-up, serum with the highest level of beta-carotene was associated with a 59 percent reduction in the diabetes risk. On the other hand, serum with the lowest concentration of beta-carotene was associated with an increased risk of developing insulin resistance.

In contrast to the above study, the analysis of a population (29,133 male smokers ages fifty to sixty-nine years) enrolled in the Alpha-Tocopherol, Beta-Carotene Cancer Prevention (ATBC) Study revealed that supplementation with beta-carotene alone did not reduce the risk of type 2 diabetes during a follow-up period of twelve and a half years (Kataja-Tuomola et al. 2008). This could be due to the fact that the high oxidative environment of the smokers may have oxidized beta-carotene, which then acts as a pro-oxidant rather than as an antioxidant.

It is interesting to note that in animal studies, supplementation with vitamin A was used to evaluate the benefit of this vitamin in reducing the development or progression of diabetes; however, none of the human survey-types of studies have evaluated the association between an intake of vitamin A and the risk of developing diabetes. Therefore, the significance of vitamin A supplementation in the prevention of diabetes remains uncertain.

Vitamin C

It has been demonstrated that an infusion of vitamin C blocked acute hyperglycemia-induced damage to endothelial cells in adolescents with type 1 diabetes (Hoffman et al. 2012).

Vascular endothelial dysfunction (a defect in the capacity of blood vessels to dilate) and increased arterial intima media thickness (IMT:

thickness of artery walls) contribute to the development of heart disease in type 1 diabetes. Since increased oxidative stress is involved in causing endothelial dysfunction and increased IMT, the importance of plasma levels of vitamins was correlated with endothelial dysfunction and increased IMT. The results showed that lower plasma levels of vitamins were associated with the increased IMT and endothelial dysfunction, suggesting that supplementation with vitamin C may improve endothelial dysfunction and prevent an increase in IMT in patients with type 1 diabetes (Odermarsky et al. 2009).

In a review of fifteen survey-types of studies involving 4,094 individuals, it was found that dietary intake or plasma levels of vitamin C were not associated with diabetes-related retinopathy (damage to the eyes) (Lee et al. 2010).

In a survey-type of study in Europe (the European Prospective Investigation of Cancer-Norfolk) involving 21,831 individuals ages forty to seventy-five at baseline, it was found that high plasma levels of vitamin C, and to a lesser extent fruit and vegetable intake, were associated with a decreased risk of diabetes (Harding et al. 2008).

The results from these studies on vitamin C and the risk of diabetes have been inconsistent.

Vitamin D$_3$

Epidemiologic studies have supported the role of vitamin D$_3$ in reducing the risk of developing diabetes. An epidemiologic study involving patients with prediabetes revealed that higher plasma levels of vitamin D$_3$ were associated with a lower risk of developing type 2 diabetes (Pittas et al. 2012).

In another epidemiology study performed in Norway, plasma levels of vitamin D$_3$ were measured in the following patient groups:

1. One thousand one hundred ninety-three patients with normal glucose tolerance
2. Three hundred four patients with impaired fasting glucose

3. Two hundred fifty-four patients with impaired glucose tolerance
4. One hundred thirty-nine patients with a combination of impaired fasting glucose and impaired glucose tolerance
5. One hundred ninety-four patients with type 2 diabetes

The results showed that higher levels of serum vitamin D_3 were associated with an improvement in glucose metabolism and insulin sensitivity compared to normal subjects (Hutchinson et al. 2011).

A deficiency in vitamin D_3 may increase the risk of type 2 diabetes. This was supported by several studies. Vitamin D_3 deficiency was found among obese children and adolescents (Buyukinan et al. 2012), but it was more prevalent in type 2 diabetes than in type 1 diabetes (Nwosu et al. 2012).

In an epidemiologic study performed in Australia, it was found that vitamin D_3 deficiency was associated with an increased risk of metabolic syndrome (Gagnon et al. 2012). These studies suggest that supplementation with vitamin D_3 could be useful in the management of diabetes.

Vitamin E

In a review of fifteen studies involving 4,094 individuals, it was found that dietary intake or plasma levels of vitamin E were not associated with diabetes-related retinopathy (damage to the eyes) (Lee et al. 2010).

In a Swedish clinical study (Uppsala Longitudinal Study of Adult Men) involving 846 non-diabetic fifty-year-old men, the serum concentration of alpha-tocopherol was correlated with insulin resistance and type 2 diabetes (Arnlov et al. 2009). The results showed that during twenty-seven years of follow-up, the serum with the highest level of alpha-tocopherol was associated with a 46 percent reduction in diabetes risk. On the other hand, serum with the lowest concentration of alpha-tocopherol was associated with an increased risk of developing insulin resistance.

The results of these studies on vitamin E and diabetes risk have been inconsistent.

Multiple Antioxidants

Using an epidemiologic (survey-type) study involving a total of 232,007 individuals (14,130 individuals with diabetes and 217,877 individuals with no diabetes), the effectiveness of multivitamins in reducing the risk of diabetes was evaluated (Song et al. 2011). Three commercial types of multivitamin preparations—Stresstabs, Theragran, and once-a-day vitamins were used. Multivitamin use was assessed by a food-frequency questionnaire at baseline from 1995–1996. The cases of diabetes that were diagnosed after the year 2000 were included in the analysis of the results. The results showed that consumption of multivitamins was not associated with a reduction in the risk of developing type 2 diabetes. Considering the involvement of oxidative stress in the development of type 2 diabetes, this finding was surprising. The authors of this survey suggested that the doses of antioxidants present in the multivitamins may not have been sufficient to decrease oxidative stress and inflammation, and certain ingredients present in the multivitamins may have been nullifying the antioxidant effect of the multivitamins.

In my opinion, the above-cited study does not allow one to make any valid conclusions regarding the value of multivitamins in reducing the risk of diabetes. This matter can be resolved only if a *full* complement of vitamins containing dietary and endogenous antioxidants, B vitamins, vitamin D_3, and certain minerals is administered orally every day by a population at high risk for developing diabetes, for at least a five-year period. The markers of oxidative stress and inflammation as well as the risk of developing diabetes should also be determined.

Omega-3 Fatty Acids

A recent review of several epidemiologic studies showed that dietary intake of fish/seafood or EPA + DHA had no effect on the risk of developing type 2 diabetes; however, higher levels of ALA (omega-3 fatty acids derived from plants) may be associated with a reduced risk of diabetes (Wu et al. 2012).

Some studies have suggested that populations consuming large amounts of omega-3 fatty acids found mainly in fish reduced the incidence of impaired glucose tolerance, type 2 diabetes, and cardiovascular disease. This was not confirmed by another large epidemiologic study, which involved 195,000 adults in the United States (152,700 women and 42,500 men) without pre-existing chronic disease at baseline with a follow-up period of fourteen to eighteen years. The results showed that a higher consumption of omega-3 fatty acids and fish was not associated with a reduced risk of type 2 diabetes. Instead, it was modestly associated with an increased incidence of the disease (Kaushik et al. 2009).

In another study involving 36,328 women, it was found that a higher intake of omega-3 fatty acids (0.20 grams/day or more, or two servings of fish/day) from marine sources but not from plant sources increased the risk of type 2 diabetes (Djousse et al. 2011b).

In contrast, the highest plasma concentrations of ALA were associated with a lower risk of diabetes (Djousse et al. 2011a). This study suggests that supplementation with omega-3 fatty acids from fish may not have an impact on the incidence of type 2 diabetes or it may even increase the risk of diabetes. On the other hand, an intake of ALA may reduce the risk of diabetes. However, this suggestion needs to be confirmed by intervention studies before it is accepted.

In an epidemiologic study performed among middle-aged Chinese men (51,963) and women (64,193), it was found that higher intakes of fish, shellfish, and omega-3 fatty acids were associated with a reduced risk of type 2 diabetes in women. However, in men, only the intake of shellfish was associated with a reduced risk of type 2 diabetes (Villegas et al. 2011).

In another study performed among Chinese men and women in Singapore, it was found that a higher intake of omega-3 fatty acids from seafood was not associated with a lower risk of type 2 diabetes, but a higher intake of omega-3 fatty acids from plants was associated with a lower risk of type 2 diabetes (Brostow et al. 2011).

Aspirin

An epidemiologic study involving 22,071 healthy men taking aspirin for a period of twenty-two years revealed that the incidence of type 2 diabetes decreased by about 14 percent (Hayashino et al. 2009) in this group. Although the decrease in the incidence of type 2 diabetes after aspirin intake was small, the results are very impressive because aspirin, which reduces inflammation but does not affect oxidative stress (one of the important events that contribute to the risk of type 2 diabetes), can decrease the incidence of this disease.

This observation needs to be confirmed by intervention studies. We will explore this further in the next chapter.

CONCLUDING REMARKS

Animal studies are useful to ascertain whether or not a particular agent has the potential to reduce the risk of developing diabetes and diabetes-related complications. Animal models of diabetes are also useful in demonstrating the involvement of biochemical and genetic factors that may be involved in the development and progression of this disease.

The animal studies discussed in this chapter also reveal that—in addition to antioxidant use—the individual and consistent use of B vitamins, vitamin D_3, L-carnitine, and omega-3 fatty acids derived from fish and plant sources, as well as aspirin, produced some beneficial effects in reducing the risk of developing diabetes. In addition, such treatments also reduced plasma glucose levels, and improved insulin sensitivity to glucose and blood-vessel function.

Although these animal studies produced some consistent results on the effectiveness of the above nutrients in reducing the risk and progression of diabetes, the results of clinical studies with the same nutrients in humans varied from no effect, to some transient beneficial effects, depending upon the type of population, type and number of vitamins and antioxidants, clinical outcomes, and period of study. The reasons for the inconsistent results in humans include (a) a failure to consider the presence of high oxidative and inflammatory environments in the high-risk patients selected for the study, (b) by and large, the use of only one nutrient at a time, (c) a lack of consideration of the form, type, dose, and dose schedule of the nutrients chosen, and (d) variations in markers of oxidative damage and inflammation from one study to another. Animal studies can be useful for showing whether or not a particular vitamin is useful in diabetes prevention or management.

No studies have been performed to evaluate the effectiveness of a full complement of dietary and endogenous antioxidants, B vitamins, and the appropriate minerals on the risk of developing type 1 and/or type 2 diabetes. As we will discuss later in the book, this author believes that the number and combination of antioxidants historically used in these studies has not been sufficient.

In the next chapter we will examine the results of a different type of study: the intervention study. As noted earlier, intervention studies tend to be more definitive than epidemiologic studies. In the ensuing discussion we will again seek to answer our most pressing questions about the role of supplements in the prevention and mitigation of the damaging effects of the disease of diabetes.

6 The Search for Prevention Part 2

The Intervention Studies

Animal and human epidemiologic studies have shown the possibility of a beneficial effect of some individual antioxidants in reducing the risk of diabetes, but the results have been inconsistent and certainly cannot be considered optimal. Therefore, it has been essential to perform intervention studies to determine the effectiveness of supplementary antioxidants, B vitamins, omega-3 fatty acids, certain minerals, aspirin, and herbs in reducing the risk of diabetes in humans.

We will discuss the results of some of these studies in this chapter. Before doing that, however, let's look at the design of a typical intervention study and examine some factors to consider when constructing one.

THE DESIGN OF AN INTERVENTION STUDY

In a typical clinical intervention study, the participating patients are divided into two groups. One group receives vitamin supplement pills and the other group receives placebo pills, which do not contain vitamins. The vitamin group is also called the experimental group and the placebo group is called the control group. Patients are randomly selected by the computer to receive vitamin pills or placebo pills. Studies are considered "blinded" when neither patients nor the provider of the pills know which group is receiving vitamins versus placebo pills. Only this type of study is considered reliable for developing public health recommendations by the established scientific community.

Prevention studies for diabetes have been split into two groups: those pertaining to primary prevention and those pertaining to secondary prevention. The purpose of primary prevention is to protect healthy individuals from developing diabetes. The purpose of secondary prevention is to stop or slow the progression of risk factors in those individuals who do not have type 2 diabetes and are not taking any diabetic medications, but who may have pre-diabetic conditions, hyperglycemia, or display insulin resistance. (Patients with type 1 diabetes who are on insulin can be included in secondary prevention.) Most clinical intervention studies have tested the effectiveness of antioxidants as secondary prevention; only a few studies pertaining to primary prevention are available.

Primary and secondary prevention strategies for individuals are implemented at the doctor's office or in the hospital, whereas for whole populations they can be implemented at the community, state, or national level in a top-down scenario.

Factors to Consider When Designing an Intervention Study

What are the appropriate patient populations for the study of diabetes? For a diabetes prevention study, it is important to select a population that is at high risk for developing the disease. The main reason for selecting a high-risk population is that the effectiveness of vitamin supplements on the risk of diabetes can be determined within a shorter period of time. High-risk populations include pre-diabetic patients, individuals with insulin resistance, obese individuals, and individuals with a family history of diabetes. In published studies on antioxidants and diabetes, the types of populations examined have varied markedly from one clinical study to another. This is one of the reasons for the inconsistent results that have contributed to confusion about the value of antioxidants in reducing the risk of diabetes.

What are blood levels of markers of oxidative stress and chronic inflammation in patients selected for the study? Populations at high risk for developing diabetes have a high internal oxidative and inflammatory environment, which should be measured at the beginning of the study. This provides an opportunity to evaluate the effectiveness of vitamin supplements in reducing the important markers of oxidative stress and inflammation. In addition, *several* markers of oxidative stress and chronic inflammation exist, but studies typically measure only one or two of them. This may not be sufficient to show the involvement of these biological processes in the development and progression of diabetes.

How many vitamins and antioxidants (single vs. multiple) should be used in the proposed study? This is a very important issue that has been ignored in most clinical studies. Although laboratory and human epidemiologic studies have shown that single antioxidants may be useful in reducing the risk of diabetes, the use of individual antioxidants in intervention studies in high-risk populations has produced transient benefits, or no effects, or even harmful effects.

This is due to the fact that a single antioxidant such as vitamin E or beta-carotene, when administered to individuals with a high internal oxidative environment, is oxidized and as such, acts as a pro-oxidant (as a free radical) rather than as an antioxidant. The continued presence of increased amounts of pro-oxidants would be ineffective after a short period of antioxidant treatment, or it would increase the risk of developing diabetes in high-risk populations subsequent to long-term consumption. If, however, the same antioxidant is present in a multivitamin preparation, the presence of other antioxidants would prevent the conversion of the administered antioxidant to a pro-oxidant.

What form, type, dose, and dose-schedule of vitamins and antioxidants should be used in the proposed study? Selection of the *form* of the respective antioxidant is important in determining its effectiveness in reducing the risk of diabetes. For example, the natural form of vitamin E (d-) accumulated in various organs of rats more than the synthetic form (dl-) of vitamin E did, following administration of both forms at the same time (Ingold et al. 1987). D-alpha-tocopheryl succinate was found to be the most effective form of vitamin E (Prasad et al. 2003).

The natural form of beta-carotene is more effective than its synthetic form in reducing the incidence of cancer in cell cultures (Kennedy and Krinsky 1994). Most major clinical studies have utilized the synthetic form of vitamin E or beta-carotene. Vitamin E (d-), alpha-tocopheryl succinate has never been used in any clinical study.

The selection of the *type* of antioxidant is also important in determining the effectiveness of antioxidants in reducing the risk of diabetes. Most clinical studies have utilized only dietary (exogenous) antioxidants such as vitamins A, C, E, beta-carotene, and selenium. Although the endogenous antioxidants such as alpha-lipoic acid, n-acetylcysteine, coenzyme Q10, and L-carnitine have been utilized, a *combination* of endogenous and exogenous dietary antioxidants has seldom been used in intervention studies. Both dietary and endogenous antioxidants regulate cellular function in part by different pathways, and they are distributed differently within the cells and among the organs. Therefore, it is essential to include both exogenous dietary and endogenous antioxidants in a multivitamin preparation that is being considered for use in a clinical study to evaluate the effectiveness of vitamins and antioxidants in reducing the risk of diabetes.

The dose and dose-schedule are also important in determining the effectiveness of antioxidants in reducing the risk of diabetes. Considering that high doses of vitamin A (10,000 IU/day or more) may produce harmful effects, the use of a lower dose of vitamin A (3,000 IU/day) is recommended. Lower doses of multiple antioxidants may only reduce oxidative damage, whereas *higher (non-toxic)* doses of antioxidants may reduce both free radicals and inflammation.

Generally, most clinical studies have utilized a dose-schedule of antioxidant supplements taken once a day. This dose-schedule may not produce an optimal effect because the biological half-lives of vitamins and antioxidants in plasma vary markedly, depending upon the extent of their solubility in water or fat, and their rate of elimination from the body. Taking a multivitamin preparation once a day may create large fluctuations in the levels of vitamins and antioxidants.

For example, a twofold change in the treatment dose of alpha-tocopheryl succinate caused marked alterations in the expression of gene profiles of neuroblastoma cells in culture (Prasad et al. 2003). This finding suggests that large fluctuations in the levels of antioxidants in the cells may force them to constantly adjust their genetic activity, which can cause cellular stress over a long period of time. Therefore, the once-a-day dose-schedule may not produce an optimal beneficial effect; however, taking a micronutrient preparation containing dietary and endogenous antioxidants twice a day might.

What type of end-points (clinical outcomes and markers of oxidative stress and chronic inflammation) should be measured at the end of the study? In all clinical studies with antioxidants, the clinical outcomes markedly differ from one study to another. Some studies have utilized clinical markers of diabetes whereas others have utilized biochemical risk markers associated with increased chances of developing diabetes.

The major primary clinical outcomes in previous studies on antioxidants and diabetes include the following:

1. Plasma glucose level
2. Insulin resistance
3. Diabetes-related complications
4. Plasma glycated hemoglobin (HbA1c) level

The major biochemical marker risk factors of diabetes in previous clinical studies on antioxidants include the following:

1. Endothelial dysfunction (abnormal blood-vessel function)
2. C-reactive protein (CRP)
3. Markers of oxidative stress
4. Pro-inflammatory cytokines

How long should the period of study be in order for it to yield meaningful results? In previous clinical studies on antioxidants and diabetes, the period of study is generally short (a few months). The period of study depends upon the selected clinical outcomes. If the clinical outcomes are markers of oxidative stress and inflammation, a shorter study period would be sufficient; however, if the clinical outcomes are major symptoms of diabetes, an observation period of at least two years is needed. The differences in clinical outcomes and study period varied from one study to another are some of the reasons for the inconsistent results that have contributed to confusion about the value of antioxidants in reducing the risk of diabetes.

SELECTED CLINICAL INTERVENTION STUDIES WITH MICRONUTRIENTS

Selected clinical studies on the effectiveness of antioxidants, the B vitamins folic acid (B₉) and thiamine (B₁), omega-3 fatty acids, chromium, aspirin, and herbs on the risk of developing diabetes are described here. As with the studies presented in the previous chapter, most of these studies utilize only one supplemental agent.

Vitamin C

In a randomized clinical study involving thirty-six elderly patients with type 2 diabetes, a dose-dependent increase in the cellular levels of reduced glutathione and vitamin E was observed after treatment with vitamin C (500 milligrams/day or 1,000 milligrams/day), compared to those who received placebo pills. These changes were not sufficient in reducing LDL susceptibility to oxidation (Tessier et al. 2009). This study was not sufficient to make any conclusion regarding the value of vitamin C alone in type 2 diabetes.

Endothelial dysfunction is associated with hyperglycemia-induced type 2 diabetes, which may become aggravated in patients with insulin resistance. In twenty subjects who had type 2 diabetes with moderate glycemic control, the effect of vitamin C alone on endothelial dysfunction was studied. The results showed that both intra-arterial and oral administration of high-dose vitamin C—1,000 milligrams/day for two days prior to testing following the ingestion of high-fat meals—improved plasma vitamin C levels, reduced endothelial dysfunction, and insulin resistance in diabetic patients (Anderson et al. 2006).

This study suggests that vitamin C supplementation may improve the symptoms of type 2 diabetes. However, the number of patients was too small to make any definite conclusion.

Vitamin D

The incidence of type 2 diabetes is higher among African Americans than it is among Caucasian Americans. This could be due to lower levels of plasma vitamin D_3 in the African Americans. In order to examine the role of vitamin D in reducing the risk of developing type 2 diabetes, the effects of 4,000 IU of vitamin D on glucose levels and insulin secretion was tested in eighty-nine overweight or obese African Americans with prediabetes or early diabetes. The results showed that supplemental vitamin D corrected vitamin D deficiency, but it decreased insulin sensitivity, increased insulin secretion, and had no effect on glucose metabolism.

Several epidemiologic studies have suggested that deficiency of vitamin D is associated with an increased risk of developing type 2 diabetes. However, well-designed clinical studies to evaluate the role of vitamin D in reducing the risk of type 2 diabetes have not been performed.

Vitamin E

Diabetes is associated with an increased risk of complications following coronary bypass graft, in which increased oxidative stress and pro-inflammatory markers and adhesion molecules play an important role. The efficacy of vitamin E in combination with standard care on markers of oxidative damage, pro-inflammatory cytokines, and adhesion molecules in diabetic patients with coronary bypass grafts was evaluated. The results showed that supplementation with vitamin E reduced oxidative stress, inflammation markers, and adhesion molecules (Hamdy et al. 2009).

The analysis of a population (29,133 male smokers ages fifty to sixty-nine) enrolled in the Alpha-Tocopherol, Beta-Carotene Cancer Prevention Study (ATBC) revealed that supplementation with alpha-tocopherol alone did not reduce the risk of type 2 diabetes during a follow-up period of twelve and one-half years (Kataja-Tuomola et al. 2008). Similar results were obtained with vitamin C, tocotrienol, and flavonols, using the same population of male smokers. This effect could be due to the fact that vitamin E—or any individual antioxidant in the presence of the high oxidative environment of the smokers—may become oxidized and act as a pro-oxidant rather than as an antioxidant.

The Women's Antioxidant Cardiovascular Study involved 8,171 female health-care professionals with either a history of cardiovascular disease or other cardiovascular risk factors. In this study, the effectiveness of vitamin C (ascorbic acid, 500 milligrams/day), vitamin E (RRR-alpha-tocopheryl acetate, 600 IU/every other day), and beta-carotene (50 milligrams/every other day)—or their respective placebos—was evaluated with respect to the risk of developing type 2 diabetes. The result showed that none of these antioxidants, when used individually, was effective in reducing the risk of type 2 diabetes (Song et al. 2009b).

Although the selection of a high-risk population for type 2 diabetes was useful, the use of only one dietary antioxidant was not. Inconsistent results with a single antioxidant have been obtained with other chronic diseases including cancer, heart disease, and neurological diseases.

Therefore, the above results were not unexpected. In any event, none of these findings should be considered to be relevant to the potential effectiveness of a vitamin preparation containing multiple dietary and endogenous antioxidants.

A Combination of Vitamins C and E

In a clinical study in the United Kingdom involving women with type 1 diabetes before pregnancy, the oral administration of 1,000 milligrams of vitamin C and 400 IU of vitamin E (alpha-tocopherol) daily during their entire pregnancy did not reduce the risk of developing preeclampsia (gestational hypertension) (McCance et al. 2010). This suggests that increased oxidative stress may not be involved in the development of preeclampsia.

In the Myocardial Infarction and Vitamins Study involving 800 patients with acute myocardial infarction (AMI) in which 122 patients (15 percent) had confirmed diabetes, the efficacy of vitamin E and vitamin C on mortality was evaluated. The results revealed that supplementation with vitamin E and vitamin C reduced heart-related mortality in patients with AMI and diabetes (Jaxa-Chamiec et al. 2009).

In a clinical study involving sixteen patients with type 2 diabetes, it was observed that supplementation with tablets containing 1,000 milligrams of vitamin C and 800 IU of vitamin E reduced high-fat-induced memory impairment and markers of oxidative stress (Chui and Greenwood 2008).

Administration of vitamin C (1,000 milligrams/day) and vitamin E (1,000 milligrams/day) for a period of four weeks decreased markers of inflammation (TNF-alpha) and oxidative damage (8-isoprostane), reduced glucose levels, and improved insulin action (Rizzo et al. 2008).

Alpha-lipoic Acid

A recent review on the role of alpha-lipoic acid in the management of type 2 diabetes has shown that alpha-lipoic acid produced beneficial effects in diabetic patients by improving the uptake and utilization of glucose (Poh and Goh 2009; Singh and Jialal 2008). Alpha-lipoic acid also reduced oxidative stress and the formation of advanced glycation end-products (AEGs) and improved insulin sensitivity to glucose in skeletal muscle and liver.

In a clinical study involving 1,500 patients with type 1 and type 2 diabetes, the effectiveness of an alpha-lipoic acid supplement in reducing damage to nerve cells was evaluated. The results showed that supplementation with alpha-lipoic acid (600 milligrams/day administered intravenously over three weeks) significantly improved nerve-cell function in patients with type 2 diabetes (Liu et al. 2007; Ziegler et al. 2006), as well as in patients with type 1 diabetes (Tankova et al. 2004).

In another clinical study, an oral administration of alpha-lipoic acid (600 milligrams/twice a day; or 600 milligrams, 1,200 milligrams, or 1,800 milligrams/once a day) increased insulin sensitivity to glucose and improved the function of nerve cells in patients with type 2 diabetes (Jacob et al. 1999; Ziegler et al. 2006).

Several other studies have demonstrated that a combination of exercise and alpha-lipoic acid produced better improvement of insulin sensitivity to glucose in skeletal muscle than either agent alone (Henriksen 2006).

In a clinical study involving thirty-two diabetic patients with retinopathy, the effect of alpha-lipoic acid (400 milligrams/day), together with genistein and vitamins, was evaluated. The results showed that an oral supplementation with antioxidants reduced damage to the eyes (Nebbioso et al. 2012).

Platelet activity is critical for preventing blood loss following an injury. However, with certain conditions such as diabetes, platelets become activated and bind with the adjacent plasma proteins to form a platelet plug that can cause a partial or full blockage of blood vessels. This phenomenon is called platelet reactivity. Type 1 diabetes is associated with increased platelet reactivity. In a clinical study involving fifty-one patients with type 1 diabetes, the effectiveness of alpha-lipoic acid (600 milligrams/day) on reducing platelet reactivity was tested.

The results showed that supplementation with alpha-lipoic acid reduced platelet reactivity in these patients compared to those who received placebo pills; however, the levels of markers of oxidative damage and inflammation were not affected by this treatment (Mollo et al. 2012). This would suggest that the beneficial effect of alpha-lipoic acid on platelet activity does not involve oxidative stress or inflammation.

In a clinical study involving fifty patients with diabetes who had deficits in both motor and sensory nerve conduction, the efficacy of alpha lipoic acid in combination with a superoxide dismutase (SOD) mimetic, ALA 600 SOD,* on improvement in sensory nerve conduction was tested. The results showed that supplementation with these antioxidants improved nerve-cell conduction (Bertolotto and Massone 2012).

In a multicenter clinical study, 233 patients with mild to moderate damage to their nerve cells received alpha-lipoic acid for four months (600 milligrams/day). Another group of 233 patients with the same condition received a placebo for the same four-month period. The results showed that alpha-lipoic acid was well tolerated and treatment with it improved the function of nerve cells (Ziegler et al. 2011) and also reduced the progression of damage to nerve cells.

A clinical study was performed in China in order to explore the effectiveness of alpha-lipoic acid on symptoms of polyneuropathy (damage to the nerve cells). The study involved 117 patients with diabetes who also displayed polyneuropathy. This group received 1,800 milligrams of alpha-lipoic acid daily for twelve weeks. Another group of 119 patients with the same disease received a placebo for the same period of time. The results showed that an oral supplementation with a high dose of alpha-lipoic acid improved symptoms of polyneuropathy.

The supplementation with alpha-lipoic acid at doses of 600 milligrams three times a day for two weeks also produced beneficial effects on the symptoms of polyneuropathy (Gu et al. 2010).

In another clinical study performed in China involving twenty-two

---

*ALA 600 SOD is the generic name of an SOD mimetic, a synthetic compound that acts like SOD.

obese individuals with impaired glucose tolerance, the administration of 600 milligrams of alpha-lipoic acid intravenously every day for two weeks improved insulin sensitivity to glucose, and decreased markers of oxidative damage and inflammation, compared to those who did not receive the alpha-lipoic acid (Zhang et al. 2011).

In a clinical study involving 102 patients with type 2 diabetes, the effectiveness of various doses of alpha-lipoic acid on lipid profiles and insulin sensitivity to glucose was determined. The results showed that supplementation with alpha-lipoic acid (600 milligrams/day) or alpha-tocopherol (800 milligrams/day) alone or in combination did not affect lipid profiles, but did enhance insulin sensitivity to glucose (de Oliveira et al. 2011). This suggested that intravenous administration of alpha-lipoic acid was very effective in improving insulin sensitivity to glucose.

Macular edema (swelling in the back of the eye) is associated with diabetes. In a clinical study involving 235 patients with type 2 diabetes, supplementation with alpha lipoic acid (600 milligrams/daily) did not prevent the occurrence of macular edema in diabetic patients compared to those who received placebo pills for a period of about nine years (Haritoglou et al. 2011).

Coenzyme Q10

In a clinical study involving twenty-eight patients with type 2 diabetes (ten men and eighteen women) and ten age-sex-matched non-diabetic individuals, the effectiveness of coenzyme Q10 in reducing the markers of oxidative stress (MDA in platelets and serum) was evaluated. The levels of MDA in platelets and serum were higher and the plasma coenzyme Q10 levels were lower in patients with diabetes than in control subjects. Higher plasma coenzyme Q10 concentrations were associated with lower glycosylated hemoglobin (Hb A1c) levels. This suggests that the patients with type 2 diabetes have a high internal oxidative environment, which may cause impaired glycemic (blood level of glucose) control in diabetic patients (El-ghoroury et al. 2009).

Maternally inherited diabetes mellitus and deafness (MIDD) is due to a mutation (defect) in mitochondrial DNA (mtDNA), and is characterized by progressive insulin secretory deficiency and neurosensory deafness. In a clinical study involving twenty-eight MIDD patients, seven patients had impaired glucose tolerance (IGT) and fifteen patients had normal glucose tolerance (NGT).* In this study, the efficacy of coenzyme Q10 (150 milligrams/day for a period of three years) on insulin secretory response, hearing disorders, and the clinical symptoms of MIDD were evaluated. The results showed that the insulin secretory response in MIDD patients was significantly higher in the treated patients than in control MIDD patients (Suzuki et al. 1998).

Coenzyme Q10 treatment also reduced the symptoms of hearing loss; however, it did not affect diabetes-related complications or other clinical symptoms of MIDD. Furthermore, coenzyme Q10 treatment did not affect insulin secretory response in those patients who showed IGT or NGT. There were no toxic effects of coenzyme Q10 during the therapy period of three years.

In a clinical study involving thirty individuals with metabolic syndrome and inadequate control of high blood pressure, the effectiveness of orally administered coenzyme Q10 (100 milligrams/twice daily for a period of twelve weeks) on high blood pressure was tested. The results showed that supplemented coenzyme Q10 did not improve high blood pressure in these patients (Young et al. 2012). Thus, the results of coenzyme Q10 alone produced variable benefits, depending on the criteria of clinical outcome measures.

L-carnitine

L-carnitine is synthesized from lysine and methionine primarily in the liver and kidneys. It plays an important role in lipid metabolism. It transports fatty acids to the mitochondria for degradation. It also plays a key role in glucose metabolism. Any reduction in the transport of fatty acids into the mitochondria can lead to the accumulation of

---

*Six patients may have dropped out of the study.

triglycerides, which contributes to insulin resistance. Indeed, it has been reported that treatment with L-carnitine and acetyl-L-carnitine improved insulin sensitivity to glucose in non-diabetic subjects as well as in patients with type 2 diabetes (Mingrone 2004).

A review of two clinical trials involving 1,679 patients with diabetes revealed that a dose of 2 grams of L-carnitine daily was well tolerated, and caused a reduction in the level of pain. One study showed improvements in nerve conduction, while the other did not (Evans et al. 2008). Evidence of nerve regeneration was found in another trial (Sima 2007).

The results of these investigations suggest that supplementation with high-dose L-carnitine may reduce some of the symptoms of diabetes-related damage to nerve cells.

Type 2 diabetes is associated with increased levels of oxidized LDL. In a randomized, placebo-controlled trial involving eighty-one patients with type 2 diabetes, supplementation with L-carnitine reduced the levels of oxidized LDL (Malaguarnera et al. 2009). Obese patients with insulin resistance to glucose have elevated levels of free fatty acids, which contribute to endothelial dysfunction. In a clinical study involving seven non-diabetic, non-obese subjects, supplementation with L-carnitine reduced the endothelial dysfunction that was associated with free fatty acids (Shankar et al. 2004).

The role of L-carnitine in diabetes is further supported by the fact that the mean serum-free L-carnitine levels in diabetic patients with complications were almost 25 percent lower than in diabetic patients without complications (Poorabbas et al. 2007).

It has been reported that a higher concentration of L-carnitine in the blood did not reduce the risk of diabetes-related complications such as retinopathy, nephropathy, and neuropathy (Liepinsh et al. 2012).

It should be noted that no supplementation of L-carnitine was used in this study; therefore, the value of L-carnitine in reducing the risk of developing diabetes-related complications cannot be determined by this study.

In type 2 diabetes, oral administration of L-carnitine (2 grams/twice daily) in combination with a calorically restricted diet reduced insulin resistance to glucose and decreased fasting glucose levels (Molfino et al. 2010).

An oral supplementation with acetyl-L-carnitine (1 gram twice daily for a period of twenty-four weeks) lowered hypertension and reduced insulin resistance to glucose in patients with type 2 diabetes with an increased risk of developing heart disease (Ruggenenti et al. 2009).

N-acetylcysteine (NAC)

In a clinical study involving ten patients with type 2 diabetes and ten non-diabetic subjects, the effect of NAC on markers of oxidative stress and chronic inflammation after a high-glucose meal was evaluated. The results showed that the levels of markers of oxidative damage (4-hydroxynonenal [HNE] and malondialdehyde [MDA]) increased after the consumption of a high-glucose meal in patients with diabetes who did not receive NAC. The glycemic index (glucose control) markers of inflammation and insulinemia (excess insulin present in the plasma) remained unchanged. However, in diabetic patients receiving a high-glucose meal after NAC administration, the levels of HNE, MDA, and the vascular adhesion molecule-1 (VCAM-1) decreased. The control subjects receiving a high-glucose meal before or after NAC administration did not show any significant change on any markers of oxidative stress or inflammation (Masha et al. 2009).

It has been reported that the blood levels of glutathione are significantly reduced in patients with type 1 diabetes; however, supplementation with low levels of cysteine, a precursor of glutathione, failed to restore glutathione levels in patients with poorly controlled type 1 diabetes (Darmaun et al. 2008).

This is in contrast to animal studies in which supplementation with high doses of L-cysteine can lower the glycemic index and markers of vascular inflammation (Jain et al. 2009).

Increased levels of the vascular cell-adhesion molecule-1 (VCAM-1) are found in patients with type 2 diabetes. This increase in the level of VCAM-1 contributes to the progression of vascular damage in this disease. Treatment of patients with type 2 diabetes with NAC (1,200 milligrams/day) reduced the vascular cell-adhesion molecule-1 (VCAM-1) compared to those who received placebo pills, suggesting that NAC treatment may slow the progression of damage to blood vessels that is inherent in individuals with diabetes (De Mattia et al. 1998).

Multiple Antioxidants

In a clinical study involving forty-six patients with type 2 diabetes, forty-six subjects with impaired glucose tolerance (IGT), and forty-six control subjects, the effectiveness of a mixture of antioxidants (vitamin E, vitamin C, and n-acetylcysteine) on markers of oxidative stress and inflammation was evaluated. The results showed that the plasma levels of markers of oxidative stress (MDA, 4-hydroxynonenal, and oxidized LDL), markers of the abnormal functioning of blood-vessel function, and the vascular adhesion molecule-1 (VCAM-1)—a marker of inflammation—were increased in all groups before supplementation with the antioxidants. However, after antioxidant supplementation, the levels of these markers (of oxidative stress and inflammation) were reduced (Neri et al. 2005) compared to those who did not receive the same supplements.

In a clinical study involving thirty patients with type 2 diabetes, it was observed that supplementation with chromium (1,000 micrograms) alone or in combination with vitamin C (1,000 milligrams) and vitamin E (800 IU) reduced oxidative stress and improved glucose metabolism (Lai 2008).

None of the above studies have utilized a full complement of dietary (exogenous) and endogenous antioxidants. Therefore, the value of multiple antioxidants in reducing the risk of developing type 2 diabetes remains to be determined.

B Vitamins: Folic Acid (B₉) and Thiamine (B₁)

Patients with type 1 diabetes have a reduced number of endothelial progenitor cells in the inner walls of blood vessels and exhibit impaired blood-vessel function. Reduced nitric oxide (NO) and increased oxidative stress contribute to the loss of endothelial cells and blood-vessel dysfunction. The analysis of gene expression profiles of endothelial cells from patients with type 1 diabetes revealed marked alterations in the expressions of 1,591 genes involved in processes regulating development, cell communication, cell adhesion, and localization compared to non-diabetic control subjects. Supplementation with folic acid alone normalized gene expression profiles in diabetic patients (van Oostrom et al. 2009). This is a remarkable observation in that treatment of patients with type 1 diabetes with a single micronutrient can restore alterations in gene expression profiles to a normal level.

In the Women's Antioxidants and Folic Acid Cardiovascular Study, which involved 5,442 female health-care professionals with a history of cardiovascular disease or women who had one or more cardiovascular disease risk factors, the effectiveness of a mixture of 2.5 milligrams of folic acid, 50 milligrams of vitamin B_6, and 1 milligram of vitamin B_{12} on reducing the risk of type 2 diabetes was evaluated. The results showed that lowering homocysteine levels by the administration of B vitamins in women with a high risk for cardiovascular disease did not reduce the risk of type 2 diabetes (Song et al. 2009a).

In a clinical study involving fifty-five type 1 diabetic patients ages five to twenty, the effectiveness of folic acid (5 milligrams/day for a period of eight weeks) on blood-vessel function was evaluated. The results showed that the levels of vascular cell adhesion molecule (VCAM) and microalbuminuria (small amounts of albumin in the urine) decreased after treatment with folic acid; however, the levels of HbA1c, intracellular adhesion molecule (ICAM), and the Von Willebrand factor (vWF)* did not significantly change compared to control groups (Alian et al. 2012).

The above study suggests that supplementation with folic acid

---

*vWF is a large glycoprotein produced by the cells of blood vessels. It mediates platelet adhesion to damaged blood-vessel cells, which is the first step in the formation of a clot.

improves endothelial function, which is impaired in type 1 diabetes.

Another clinical study involving fifty-nine patients with type 1 diabetes showed that supplementation with a high dose (300 milligrams/day) of benfotiamine, a synthetic form of thiamine (B_1), for a period of twenty-four months had no significant effect on nerve function and markers of inflammation (Fraser et al. 2012).

In a clinical study involving sixty-eight men with type 2 diabetes, supplementation with folic acid (5 milligrams/day) for a period of eight weeks decreased the levels of plasma homocysteine and serum malondialdehyde (MDA), and increased the levels of serum total antioxidant capacity (TAC), folate, and vitamin B_{12} compared to those who did not receive folic acid (control group) (Aghamohammadi et al. 2011).

Increased levels of homocysteine are frequently observed in patients with diabetic nephropathy (kidney disease). Since B-vitamin therapy decreases levels of homocysteine, the effectiveness of this therapy on kidney function (glomerular filtration rate, a measure of kidney function) in patients with type 1 and type 2 diabetes with nephropathy was tested. The results showed that supplementation with folic acid (2.5 milligrams/day), vitamin B_6 (25 milligrams/day), and vitamin B_{12} (1 milligram/day) decreased plasma homocysteine levels and improved kidney function (House et al. 2010).

The administration of thiamine (150 milligrams/day) for thirty days reduced the levels of glucose and leptin (a small hormone produced by fat cells to regulate body fat); however, markers of inflammation did not change compared to the control group (Gonzalez-Ortiz et al. 2011). The results suggest that thiamine can reduce the level of glucose without affecting the levels of markers of chronic inflammation.

Omega-3 Fatty Acids

In a clinical study involving 162 healthy individuals it was found that a moderate supplementation with fish oil did not affect insulin sensitivity to glucose, insulin secretion from beta-cells, beta-cell function, or glucose tolerance (Giacco et al. 2007).

In a clinical study involving ninety-seven patients with type 2 diabetes and no heart disease, it was found that supplementation with fish oil (4 grams/day for twelve weeks) did not improve blood-vessel function, but improved renal function without changes in blood pressure, inflammation, or oxidative stress (Wong et al. 2010).

In another clinical study involving 2,399 pregnant women, it was found that supplementation with DHA-enriched fish oil (800 milligrams/day) in the second half of pregnancy did not reduce the risk of gestational diabetes or preeclampsia compared to those pregnant women who received the same amount of vegetable oil (control group). In addition, this study reported that there were twelve prenatal deaths and five neonatal convulsions in the control group, but only three prenatal deaths and no neonatal convulsions in the group receiving DHA-enriched fish oil (Zhou et al. 2012).

In a clinical study involving twenty-eight patients with type 2 diabetes with low LDL cholesterol treated with statins for at least one year, supplementation with EPA (1,800 milligrams/day for a period of six months) improved blood-vessel function and decreased LDL cholesterol compared to those who received only statins (Sasaki et al. 2012).

In a clinical study involving 1,014 patients ages sixty to eighty with type 2 diabetes who had myocardial infarction (MI), supplementation with 18.6 grams of margarine/day (an additional intake of 223 milligrams EPA plus 149 milligrams DHS, and/or 1.9 grams ALA for forty months) reduced the incidence of ventricular arrhythmia (irregular heartbeat) compared to those who received placebo pills (Kromhout et al. 2011).

In a clinical study involving thirty-four patients with type 2 diabetes, it was reported that supplementation with 2 grams of purified EPA/DHA for a period of six weeks improved large and small blood-vessel function after a meal compared to those who received olive oil (no EPA/DHA) (Stirban et al. 2010).

A review of published data showed that supplementation with omega-3 fatty acids in type 2 diabetes has no significant effect on glycemic control or fasting insulin; however, it lowered triglycerides and VLDL cholesterol levels, but it may also raise LDL cholesterol (Hartweg et al. 2008).

Several intervention studies designed to evaluate the efficacy of various doses of omega-3 fatty acids on prevention and diabetes-related complications have produced inconsistent results. In a clinical study involving 454 Alaskan Eskimos, the effectiveness of omega-3 fatty acids on the incidence of cardiovascular disease was evaluated. (The average American consumes about 0.2 grams of omega-3 fatty acids per day, and Eskimos consume about three to four grams per day.) The intervention dose of omega-3 fatty acids was one to two grams per day. The results showed that there was no association between omega-3 fatty acid consumption and the presence of cardiovascular disease (Ebbesson et al. 2005).

In a systematic review of several clinical studies involving 1,075 patients with type 2 diabetes, the effects of dietary and non-dietary intake of omega-3 fatty acids on lipid profiles were evaluated. The results revealed that supplementation with omega-3 fatty acids decreased the levels of triglycerides, VLDL cholesterol, and VLDL triglycerides, but it slightly enhanced the level of LDL cholesterol. In addition, it showed a decrease in thrombogenesis (clot formation), but had no beneficial effects on cardiovascular disease risk factors such as HDL cholesterol, LDL particle size, glucose control, insulinemia (an excess of insulin in plasma), inflammatory biomarkers, and blood pressure (Hartweg et al. 2009; Hartweg et al. 2007).

In a clinical study involving thirty patients (sixteen males and fourteen females) with type 2 diabetes and high levels of triglycerides, it was found that after supplementation with omega-3 fatty acids, the levels of triglycerides, non-HDL cholesterol, C-reactive protein, and TNF-alpha were decreased, whereas the levels of HDL cholesterol increased, and there was no change in the levels of IL-6, a marker of chronic inflammation (De Luis et al. 2009).

In a clinical study involving eighty-one patients with type 2 diabetes, the effectiveness of omega-3 fatty acids on the levels of homocysteine and MDA was determined. The results revealed that supplementation with omega-3 fatty acids (3 grams/day for a period of two months) decreased the levels of homocysteine without changing the levels of MDA, fasting blood sugar, and CRP. This study again shows that supplementation with omega-3 fatty acids does not reduce glucose levels and other risk factors associated with cardiovascular disease (Pooya et al. 2009).

Supplementation with omega-3 fatty acids (3 grams/day for a period of two months) failed to alter insulin sensitivity to glucose in twenty-seven women with type 2 diabetes (Kabir et al. 2007).

In another study involving 1,770 children who were at increased risk of developing type 1 diabetes, the effectiveness of omega-3 fatty acid supplements on the risk of developing pancreatic islet autoimmunity was evaluated. The results showed that dietary intake of omega-3 fatty acids decreased the risk of developing islet autoimmunity in children at increased risk for type 1 diabetes (Norris et al. 2007). Most studies on omega-3-fatty acids suggest that supplementation with these fatty acids may improve some symptoms of diabetes.

Chromium

Chromium is a mineral that is essential to our body. A review of fifteen published clinical studies on the effectiveness of chromium picolinate (Crpic) in improving some of the markers of type 2 diabetes revealed that supplementation with Crpic reduced hyperglycemia, hyperinsulinemia (excess of plasma insulin), and need for hyperglycemic medication (Broadhurst and Domenico 2006).

In a clinical study involving patients with metabolic syndrome (obese and non-diabetic), the effectiveness of Crpic on the insulin sensitivity to glucose was evaluated. The results showed that after sixteen weeks of treatment, there were no significant changes in insulin sensitivity to glucose, body weight, serum lipids, or markers of oxidative stress and inflammation between the control group and the treated group. However, Crpic treatment increased acute insulin response to glucose (Iqbal et al. 2009). This study has no conflict with the studies above, because all of the above studies were performed on patients with type 2 diabetes. It is possible that the mechanisms of action of Crpic in diabetic patients and obese non-diabetic subjects are different.

In a clinical study involving fourteen hospitalized patients with severe insulin resistance to glucose, it was found that an infusion of chromium chloride at 20 micrograms/hour for ten to fifteen hours, for a total dose of 200 to 300 micrograms, markedly decreased glucose levels and insulin resistance to glucose in these patients (Drake et al. 2012).

In another clinical study involving forty newly diagnosed patients with type 2 diabetes, it was reported that supplementation with 9 grams of brewer's yeast containing 42 micrograms of chromium reduced blood glucose levels and total cholesterol, triglycerides, and LDL cholesterol in these patients, compared to patients who received the same dose of brewer's yeast but without chromium (Sharma et al. 2011).

A review of forty-one studies showed that chromium supplementation decreased the blood glucose level in patients with diabetes; however, it did not produce a similar effect on individuals who did not have diabetes (Balk et al. 2007).

In contrast to the above conclusion, in a clinical study involving fifty-nine adult patients with impaired fasting glucose (IFG), impaired glucose tolerance (IGT), or metabolic syndrome, supplementation with 500 or 1,000 micrograms of chromium for a period of six months did not change glucose levels, insulin levels, or insulin resistance to glucose (Ali et al. 2011).

It was suggested that a beneficial effect of chromium (a decreased glucose level and an increased insulin sensitivity to glucose) may be observed in patients with type 2 diabetes who have insulin resistance to glucose and who have elevated levels of glucose and HbA1c (Wang and Cefalu 2010).

It is interesting to note that the level of chromium in the eyes of diabetic patients with cataracts was found to be lower than in individuals with age-related cataracts (Cumurcu et al. 2008).

In contrast to chromium, chromium picolinate is fairly non-toxic. In rats, doses of chromium picolinate equaling 3,250 or 2,000 milligrams/kilogram of body weight did not produce chromosomal damage in bone marrow cells. A dose of 33 milligram/kilogram of body weight in rats is estimated to be equivalent to 200 micrograms of chromium for a 50-kilogram individual (Komorowski et al. 2008).

Aspirin and Aspirin Resistance

Patients with diabetes have a high risk of developing heart disease, and consequently low-dose aspirin is widely recommended to reduce this risk. However, supplementation with aspirin failed to reduce the risk of heart disease in patients with type 2 diabetes in some major clinical studies (Ogawa et al. 2008; Price and Holman 2009).

Although some studies have suggested some minor beneficial effects of aspirin on heart disease (Sacco et al. 2003), its continued use has been suggested by many current diabetic guidelines (Colwell 2004; Younis et al. 2009). The role of aspirin in the prevention of diabetes has become controversial.

In a clinical study involving 38,716 women free of diabetes, 19,326 received aspirin and 19,390 received placebo. After a period of ten years, the effectiveness of aspirin treatment on the incidence of type 2 diabetes was evaluated. The results showed that long-term consumption of low-dose aspirin failed to prevent the development of type 2 diabetes in non-diabetic women (Pradhan et al. 2009).

A combination of aspirin and statins increased weight loss in patients with type 2 diabetes (Boaz et al. 2009).

A review of several studies has revealed that aspirin treatment did not lower the risk of diabetic retinopathy (Bergerhoff et al. 2002).

Although aspirin has become an essential component of the treatment of cardiovascular disease associated with or without type 2 diabetes because of its anti-platelet aggregation activity, the phenomenon of aspirin-resistance has become one of great interest because of its implication in increasing the risk of serious heart-disease events.

A review of studies on aspirin has revealed that about 20–30 percent of aspirin-treated patients exhibit platelet hyperactivity despite adequate inhibition of cyclooxygenase-1 (COX-1) activity. Additionally, several reviews have suggested that the existence of platelet hyperactivity could be a risk factor for developing a reduced blood supply to the heart in aspirin-treated patients (Miyata et al. 2008; Patel and Moonis 2007; Reny et al. 2009). Thus, aspirin exhibits two contrasting functions: it can reduce the risk of heart-disease-related events and increase platelet activity, which can form a clot.

Herbs

Among the herbs, cinnamon, curcumin, and milk thistle have been studied in animals and humans as regards reducing the risk and progression of diabetes. These herbs exhibit antioxidant and anti-inflammation activities that play a role in the mitigation of diabetes. Summarizations of selected reviews and papers on this subject are described here.

Cinnamon is a rich source of polyphenolics, which have been used for centuries in Chinese medicine. Procyanidin oligomers in cinnamon are responsible for its biological activity. They reduce plasma glucose levels and improve insulin sensitivity to glucose in streptozotocin-induced diabetes in mice (Lu et al. 2011).

A comprehensive review of eight well-designed clinical studies revealed that supplementation with cinnamon extract or whole cinnamon lowers fasting glucose levels in patients with type 2 diabetes (Davis and Yokoyama 2011).

In another clinical study involving 487 patients with type 2 diabetes, it was found that supplementation with milk thistle (silybum marianum) reduced fasting blood glucose levels (Suksomboon et al. 2011).

In another clinical study, one group of twenty-five patients with type 2 diabetes received milk thistle (a 200-milligram tablet/three times a day together with conventional therapy for a period of four months), whereas a second group of twenty-five patients with diabetes received placebo pills together with conventional therapy for the same period of time. The results showed that treatment with milk thistle reduced HbA1c, fasting blood glucose levels, total cholesterol, LDL cholesterol, and triglycerides, compared to those who received placebo pills (Huseini et al. 2006).

Meriva, a preparation of curcumin, the orange pigment of turmeric, was administered to twenty-five patients with type 2 diabetes at a dose of 1 gram/day for four weeks to test its effectiveness on microangiopathy (small-vessel disease). The results showed that treatment with Meriva decreased the incidence of small-vessel disease (Appendino et al. 2011).

In a clinical study involving forty patients with type 2 diabetes with nephropathy, 500 milligrams of turmeric (containing 22.2 milligrams of curcumin, the active ingredient) was administered to twenty patients three times a day for a period of two months. The control group of twenty patients received placebo pills for the same period of time. The results showed that turmeric supplementation decreased proteinuria (an increased urine level of protein, a sign of damage to the kidneys) and some markers of inflammation (Khajehdehi et al. 2011). Studies on selected herbs suggest that they could improve some symptoms of diabetes.

CONCLUDING REMARKS

Most previous clinical studies in primary prevention have utilized one or two dietary antioxidants, whereas in secondary prevention most studies have utilized only one or a few dietary antioxidants. These clinical studies yielded inconsistent results as regards impacts on the prevention and management of diabetes. These results varied from some transient beneficial effects, to no effects, to harmful effects.

The possible reasons for these inconsistent results in all previous clinical studies include the following:

1. The use of only one, two, or three dietary or endogenous antioxidants.

2. The failure to use a micronutrient preparation containing *multiple* dietary antioxidants (vitamin A, beta-carotene, vitamin C, vitamin D, vitamin E, and the mineral selenium) and endogenous antioxidants (alpha-lipoic acid, coenzyme Q10, L-carnitine, and n-acetylcysteine, a synthetic glutathione-elevating agent).

3. The use of omega-3 fatty acids alone rather than in combination with a micronutrient preparation as described above.

4. The use of certain herbs alone rather than in combination with a micronutrient preparation as described above.

5. The failure to utilize a dose-schedule of twice a day (morning and evening) to achieve a more constant level of micronutrients in the body.

The inconsistent results achieved by the studies in this chapter underscore the need to clinically examine the potential therapeutic efficacy of a multiple-micronutrient formulation to treat and manage the debilitating disease of diabetes. In the following chapter, we will look in even closer detail at the fundamental flaws of current studies that have led to inconclusive and even misleading results.

7 Current Clinical Studies

A Flawed Methodology

Although there is a uniformity of opinion among the scientific and health-care communities about the value of changes in diet and lifestyle (such as losing weight and increased physical activity) for reducing the incidence of diabetes, there is no such consensus about the value of vitamin and antioxidant supplements.

Conflicting reports on the effects of the antioxidants, various vitamins, omega-3 fatty acids (from both plant and fish sources), and other agents previously discussed, in reducing the risk of diabetes in high-risk populations are often reported in newspapers, magazines, and Internet-based media. Even though original scientific papers report only an *association* between the intake of vitamins and the risk of diabetes, the media often gives the impression that increased antioxidant levels may be ineffective or in some cases *increase* the risk of developing diabetes. For example, one day you might read that vitamin E reduces the risk of diabetes, and another day you will read that vitamin E may increase the risk of some symptoms of this disease.

In the previous chapter we described why the clinical studies that have been done to date have failed to yield consistent, beneficial results in reducing the risk of diabetes. In this chapter we will take a closer look at this problematic situation. We will also examine why controversies about this continue to exist among many physicians and health-care professionals, and what should be done to resolve the matter.

COMPONENTS OF THE FLAWED METHODOLOGY CURRENTLY USED TO DERIVE STUDY RESULTS

In this author's view, there are several reasons why current recommendations for the prevention and treatment of diabetes are not having the desired outcomes. We will examine these factors here.

A Lack of Adherence to All of the Criteria of an Intervention Study

Much of the solution necessary to reduce the incidence of diabetes and obtain an accord among treating physicians about it might be obtained if the methodology used to derive study results were thoroughly adhered to. To examine this point in a comprehensive fashion, we will revisit the criteria for a successful intervention study as outlined in the previous chapter in order to pinpoint where the failings may lie.

Those criteria are as follows:

1. What are the appropriate patient populations for the study of diabetes?
2. What are blood levels of markers of oxidative stress and chronic inflammation in patients selected for the study?
3. How many vitamins and antioxidants (single versus multiple) should be used in the proposed study?
4. What form, type, dose, and dose-schedule of vitamins and antioxidants should be used in the proposed study?
5. What type of end-points (clinical outcomes and markers of oxidative stress and chronic inflammation) should be measured at the end of the study?
6. How long need the period of study be in order for it to yield meaningful results?

In the study designs of all previous clinical trials, questions 1, 5, and 6 were carefully considered but questions 2, 3, and 4 were not, and furthermore, were often ignored. This may have contributed to conflicting results on the effectiveness of vitamins, antioxidants, chromium, and omega-3 fatty acid supplementation in reducing the risk of diabetes. Furthermore, inconsistent results obtained from the use of a single antioxidant, B vitamin, chromium, or omega-3 fatty acids alone in individuals at high risk for developing diabetes are primarily responsible for the continued doubts about the value of vitamins and antioxidants (in reducing the risk of diabetes).

It is incorrect to think that the effects of a single *agent* on diabetes prevention or treatment would produce the same effects as those produced by a preparation of multiple-micronutrients. Nevertheless, many in the medical and scientific community believe that a multiple micronutrient preparation may produce results similar to those produced by a single micronutrient and therefore do not feel comfortable recommending a more complex preparation to their patients to reduce the risk of diabetes.

Another factor to consider is that the clinical studies done to date have relied heavily on the experimental design with respect to use of only one antioxidant in animal studies, and did not consider the consequences of the administration of a single antioxidant in the high internal oxidative environment of patients who are at a high risk for developing diabetes. These include individuals with pre-diabetes, those with insulin resistance, obese individuals, or individuals with metabolic syndrome. Let's look at this a little more closely now.

Reliance on the Results of Animal Studies for the Design of Human Studies

Animal studies have consistently shown that the administration of a single antioxidant reduced an increase in the risk of diabetes that was chemically induced, or induced via the forced consumption of a high-fat diet. From the results of these studies alone, one should not conclude that similar results with a single antioxidant would be obtained in humans. It should be always remembered that animal studies with antioxidants provide *only a guide* with respect to their effectiveness in reducing the risk of diabetes in humans. The effective dose, dose-schedule, safety, and period of observation that are used in animal studies with antioxidants cannot be used in the experimental design of human studies.

This is due to the fact that the extent of effectiveness, absorption, metabolism (turnover), excretion (elimination), and toxicity of antioxidants in animals is totally different from those in humans. In addition, most mammals (except guinea pigs) make their own vitamin C, whereas humans do not. Humans rely on their diet for vitamin C. The presence of endogenous vitamin C in most animals can influence the effectiveness of a micronutrient preparation containing multiple antioxidants in reducing the risk of diabetes. In addition, animals may not have an internal oxidative environment, and the study period is generally very short compared to human studies.

The High Internal Oxidative Environment of High-risk Populations

Most clinical studies have utilized a single dietary and endogenous antioxidant in order to evaluate its effectiveness in reducing the risk of diabetes in high-risk populations. High-risk individuals with insulin resistance, hyperglycemia, or obesity have a high internal oxidative environment. As stated earlier in this book, a single antioxidant such as vitamin E or beta-carotene, when administered in the presence of a high-oxidative environment, is gradually oxidized and would then act as a pro-oxidant (like a free radical) rather than as an antioxidant.

Based on this effect, the use of a single antioxidant in any clinical study to evaluate the effectiveness of antioxidants in reducing the risk of diabetes is not justified. If the same single antioxidant is present in a vitamin preparation containing multiple dietary and endogenous antioxidants, the conversion of an antioxidant to a pro-oxidant would not occur because other antioxidants would prevent this from happening.

THE RATIONALE FOR USING A PREPARATION CONTAINING MULTIPLE-MICRONUTRIENTS

We propose the utilization of a multivitamin preparation containing dietary and endogenous antioxidants in clinical trials designed to explore how best to prevent and improve management of diabetes. B vitamins and the appropriate minerals such as selenium and chromium should also be added to this supplement.

There are several reasons to use a multivitamin preparation in clinical studies. As we know, increased oxidative stress and chronic inflammation are important factors that participate in the development and progression of diabetes. Antioxidants reduce the levels of oxidative stress and chronic inflammation. Therefore, the use of antioxidants is essential in order to reduce these risk factors. Multiple antioxidants act in a synergistic manner in order to influence disease processes in a beneficial manner.

We know that innumerable free radicals are produced by the human body on a daily basis. The body also contains multiple dietary and endogenous antioxidants, which destroy these free radicals when they are produced in excessive amounts. Each antioxidant has a different affinity for each of these free radicals, depending upon the cellular environment. For instance, we know that the level of oxygen pressure varies within cells and tissues. We also know that vitamin E is more effective in neutralizing free radicals in an environment of reduced oxygen pressure, whereas beta-carotene and vitamin A are more effective in environments that have higher oxygen pressure environments.

Vitamin C is necessary to protect cellular components immersed in water against free radical damage, whereas carotenoids, vitamin A, and vitamin E protect cellular components in lipid (fat-soluble) environments. Vitamin C also plays an important role in maintaining cellular levels of vitamin E by recycling damaged vitamin E (oxidized) to the antioxidant (reduced) form.

The form and type of vitamin E used are also important to improve its beneficial effects. It is known that various organs of rats selectively absorb the natural form of vitamin E; therefore, the natural form of vitamin E is recommended in multivitamin preparations.

The natural form of beta-carotene is also more effective than its synthetic counterpart. To illustrate this point, we know that natural beta-carotene reduced radiation-induced cancer formation in mammalian cells in culture, but synthetic beta-carotene did not (Kennedy and Krinsky 1994).

Antioxidants are distributed differently in various organs and even within the same cells. Selenium, a co-factor of glutathione peroxidase, acts as an antioxidant. Therefore, selenium supplementation together with other dietary and endogenous antioxidants is also important.

Glutathione, an endogenously made antioxidant, is an agent that is very potent in protecting the cells of the body from oxidative damage. It catabolizes H_2O_2 and anions and is very effective in neutralizing peroxynitrite, a powerful form of free radical derived from nitrogen. Therefore, increasing intracellular levels of glutathione is essential for the protection of various components within the cells. Oral supplementation with glutathione does not significantly increase plasma levels of glutathione in humans, suggesting that this antioxidant is destroyed in the gastrointestinal tract.

N-acetylcysteine is not destroyed in the intestinal tract, and when it enters the cells, n-acetyl is removed, and cysteine is used to make glutathione. Alpha-lipoic acid, an endogenously made antioxidant, also increases the level of glutathione in cells. Therefore, in order to optimally increase the level of glutathione, it is necessary to use both n-acetylcysteine and alpha-lipoic acid in a multivitamin preparation.

Coenzyme Q10, an endogenously made antioxidant, is needed by the mitochondria to generate energy. In addition, it scavenges peroxyl radicals faster than alpha-tocopherol, and like vitamin C, can regenerate vitamin E. Therefore, the addition of coenzyme Q10 in a multivitamin preparation is important for an optimal beneficial effect as well.

A CLOSER LOOK AT
DOSES AND DOSING SCHEDULES

Doses of a single antioxidant such as vitamin C (up to 10,000 milligrams/day), vitamin E (up to 600 IU/day), vitamin D (up to 4,000 IU/day), alpha-lipoic acid (up to 600 milligrams/day), n-acetylcysteine (up to 1,200 milligrams/day), L-carnitine (up to 2 grams/day), coenzyme Q10 (up to 1,200 milligrams/day), and omega-3 fatty acids (up to 4 grams/day) were used in previous clinical studies. The doses of all ingredients in a multivitamin preparation, especially dietary and endogenous antioxidants, should be higher than RDA values, while still being safe. Higher doses of antioxidants are needed in order to inhibit oxidative stress and inflammation. (Lower doses of antioxidants may reduce oxidative stress but not chronic inflammation.) We will detail more specific recommendations for micronutrient supplements in chapter 8 of this book.

Most clinical studies have utilized a once-a-day dose-schedule; however, taking vitamins and antioxidants once a day creates large fluctuations in their levels in the body. As we have established previously in the book, this is due to the fact that the biological half-lives of vitamins and antioxidants vary markedly, depending upon their lipid or water solubility. A twofold difference in the levels of vitamin E succinate can produce marked alterations in the expression profiles of several genes in neuroblastoma cells in culture. Thus, taking a multivitamin preparation once a day may produce large fluctuation in the levels of micronutrients in the body. This could potentially cause genetic stress in cells that may compromise the effectiveness of the vitamin supplementation after long-term consumption. Therefore, I recommend taking a preparation of micronutrients containing multiple dietary and endogenous antioxidants twice a day in order to maintain a more constant level of micronutrients in the body.

Additionally, most clinical studies have utilized omega-3 fatty acids alone in order to evaluate their effectiveness in reducing the risk of diabetes. As discussed earlier, omega-3 fatty acids from plant sources occurs in the form of ALA (alpha-linolenic acid). ALA appears to be more useful than omega-3 fatty acids from fish sources in reducing the risk of diabetes; however, omega-3 fatty acids from fish sources appears to be more useful in reducing the risk of heart disease. Therefore, in addition to consuming a preparation of micronutrients, taking omega-3 fatty acids from plant sources may be important for reducing the risk of diabetes.

HOW TO RESOLVE PRESENT CONTROVERSIES REGARDING MICRONUTRIENT SUPPLEMENTATION

The inconsistent results obtained by the use of one or two dietary or endogenous antioxidants, B vitamins, vitamin D, chromium, and/or omega-3 fatty acids alone in a high-risk population suggest that such experimental designs are not sufficient to determine the effectiveness of vitamins and antioxidants in reducing the risk of diabetes. The fate of individual antioxidants in a high oxidative environment also suggests that the use of a single antioxidant may be counterproductive.

Therefore, I propose a clinical study in high-risk populations in which all six criteria, found earlier in this chapter on page 131, are included. I suggest that a multiple-micronutrient preparation containing dietary and endogenous antioxidants, B vitamins, vitamin D, and appropriate minerals such as selenium and chromium picolinate, and omega-3 fatty acids (primarily from plant sources), together with a diet low in fat and high in fiber, and changes in lifestyle, should be included in any such clinical trial. The doses of antioxidants and vitamins should be higher than RDA values, but not toxic.

The preparation of micronutrients should contain dietary and endogenous antioxidants. Dietary antioxidants include vitamin A and natural, mixed carotenoids (90 percent of mixed carotenoids represent beta-carotene), two forms of vitamin E (d-alpha-tocopheryl acetate and d-alpha-tocopheryl succinate, also called vitamin E succinate), and vitamin C (calcium ascorbate). Endogenous antioxidants include alpha-lipoic acid, n-acetylcysteine, coenzyme Q10, and L-carnitine. In addition, other ingredients include vitamin D and all of the B vitamins as well as minerals such as selenium (selenomethionine), zinc, calcium, magnesium, and chromium picolinate.

It should be noted that both vitamin A and beta-carotene were added because beta-carotene, in addition to acting as a precursor of vitamin A, performs unique functions that cannot be produced by vitamin A and vice versa. Beta-carotene is more effective in destroying oxygen radicals than most other antioxidants. Thus, the addition of both vitamin A and beta-carotene may enhance the efficacy of a micronutrient preparation in diabetes prevention.

Vitamin E succinate is now considered the most effective form of vitamin E. Vitamin E succinate (being more soluble than alpha-tocopherol or alpha-tocopheryl acetate) enters the cells more easily. Here it is converted to alpha-tocopherol and thus provides intracellular (within the cell) protection against oxidative damage. It also has its own unique function as vitamin E succinate because it alters the expression of many genes in mammalian cells in culture. Therefore, in order to increase the efficacy of vitamin E, the addition of both forms of vitamin E is important.

This recommended micronutrient preparation also contains certain herbs such as cinnamon, milk thistle, and curcumin. Although the antioxidant and anti-inflammatory effects of these herbs may be similar to those produced by dietary and endogenous antioxidants, they may produce some beneficial effects on diabetes that are not related to their effects as antioxidants. (The proposed micronutrient formulation does not contain iron, copper, or manganese, for reasons previously discussed.)

The placebo group in the proposed experimental design should not have any dietary recommendations or changes in lifestyle. Dietary and lifestyle compliance can be monitored by questionnaires, whereas the compliance for the micronutrient group can be monitored by measuring plasma (blood) levels of the selected micronutrients every six months. This will test the effectiveness of all three components together: a preparation of multivitamins, omega-3 fatty acid supplementation, and changes in the diet and lifestyle.

In a subgroup of the same high-risk population, the effectiveness of vitamins and antioxidants together with omega-3 fatty acids alone is determined by providing the placebo group with the same recommendations for changes in the diet and lifestyle as those for vitamin-omega-3 fatty acid supplement group.

The results from these studies would provide conclusive proof as to whether or not a vitamin-omega-3 fatty acid supplement together with changes in the diet and lifestyle produced more beneficial effects in reducing the risk of diabetes compared to those who received only vitamin-omega-3 fatty acid supplementation.

One may argue that the proposed design of a clinical study is complicated because at the end of the study we may not know which particular vitamin or omega-3 fatty acids or diet and lifestyle change is responsible for reducing the risk of diabetes. This argument may not be valid because the primary aim of a clinical study is to achieve success in reducing the risk of the disease. For a mechanistic study on vitamins or omega-3 fatty acids, the effects of a single antioxidant or multiple antioxidants are best studied in animal and cell-culture models.

CONCLUDING REMARKS

Despite numerous clinical studies primarily using a single antioxidant in populations at high risk for developing diabetes, controversy still exists about the usefulness of antioxidant supplements in reducing the risk of this disease. I have critically examined the results of these studies and concluded that the present trend in clinical research—using a single antioxidant or at most, a very few to evaluate the effectiveness of vitamins and antioxidants in reducing the risk of diabetes—lacks scientific rationale, and therefore, these studies have not yielded definitive results.

I have provided potential reasons for the controversies that exist at this time with respect to the usefulness of vitamins and antioxidants in diabetes prevention. I have also provided the rationale and evidence for a shift in the design of clinical studies from using one antioxidant alone, or only a scant handful, to using a multivitamin preparation containing dietary and endogenous antioxidants, B vitamins, vitamin D, appropriate minerals, and omega-3 fatty acids, together with a diet low in fat and high in fiber. Conclusive evidence about the effectiveness of micronutrients in reducing the risk of diabetes can only be established by well-designed clinical intervention studies in which a micronutrient supplement is administered orally to normal or high-risk patients, and when the incidence of diabetes is compared between the micronutrient group and the control group (those who receive a placebo pill that looks like the supplement) after a period of at least two years.

We will examine my specific recommendations in the next and final chapter of this book.

8 Diabetes Prevention and Management

Multi-micronutrients, Diet, and Lifestyle Recommendations

As we have determined, the incidence of diabetes in the world—including in the United States—is on the uptick, in spite of the prevailing recommendations currently in place. This implies that these recommendations are not having the desired results. This chapter discusses a strategy to help in the prevention of diabetes, using multiple micronutrients to supplement the prevailing recommendations. We include various tables to better assist the consumer in ascertaining which recommenced multi-micronutrient supplement is best for them. We then go on to discuss current findings and suggested multiple-micronutrient supplementation in combination with standard care.

PROPOSED RECOMMENDATIONS FOR PRIMARY PREVENTION

As we know, the purpose of primary prevention is to prevent non-diabetic individuals or pre-diabetic individuals from developing diabetes. Primary prevention strategies include recommendations to avoid exposure to those agents that can induce one or more risk factors for developing the disease.

Primary Prevention Strategies for Type 1 and Type 2 Diabetes

Primary prevention strategies for both type 1 diabetes and type 2 diabetes should be adopted from childhood. Pregnant women who have a family history of type 1 diabetes should also adopt primary prevention strategies. The formulation that these pregnant women should take before, during, and after pregnancy is provided in table 8.1 below. It should be noted that an additional supplement of 30 milligrams of iron (ferrous citrate), taken during pregnancy only, can be provided in order to prevent anemia, which occurs frequently in pregnant women. Iron supplementation can be given a few hours after taking a preparation of multiple-micronutrients.

TABLE 8.1. FORMULATION FOR PREGNANT WOMEN WITH A FAMILY HISTORY OF TYPE 1 OR PATIENTS WITH TYPE 1 DIABETES OR TYPE 2 DIABETES (18–35+ YEARS)*

Vitamin A (palmitate)	3,000 IU
Natural mixed carotenoids	15 mg
Vitamin C (as calcium ascorbate)	500 mg
Vitamin D₃ (cholecalciferol)	800 IU
Vitamin E (two forms)	200 IU d-alpha-tocopherol acetate 100 IU d-alpha-tocopheryl acid succinate 100 IU
Vitamin B₁ (thiamine mononitrate)	4 mg
Vitamin B₂ (riboflavin)	5 mg
Vitamin B₃ (as niacinamide ascorbate)	30 mg
Vitamin B₆ (pyridoxine HCl)	5 mg
Folate (folic acid)	800 mcg
Vitamin B₁₂ (as cyanocobalamin)	10 mcg

*Total capsules per day can be taken orally, half in the morning and half in the evening.

Biotin	200 mcg
Pantothenic acid (as d-calcium pantothenate)	10 mg
Calcium citrate	250 mg
Magnesium citrate	125 mg
Zinc glycinate	15 mg
Selenium (L-selenomethionine)	100 mcg
Chromium (as chromium picolinate)	50 mcg

Let's look at some other specific primary prevention strategies for both type 1 diabetes and type 2 diabetes next.

Changes in Diet and Lifestyle

Increased levels of oxidative stress and chronic inflammation are found in obese individuals and individuals with insulin resistance. Thus, dietary and lifestyle changes are very important in order to prevent obesity and the development of insulin resistance, both of which are considered major risk factors for diabetes.

Diet

I recommend the daily consumption of a low-fat, high-fiber diet with plenty of fruits (especially grapes and berries) and leafy vegetables. It is also recommended that one should avoid an excessive intake of carbohydrates or proteins. Whenever oil is used for cooking, virgin olive oil is preferred because it is rich in alpha-linolenic acid, which has been shown to produce beneficial effects in patients with diabetes. For non-vegetarians, fish (especially salmon) twice a week, and chicken (or another meat not to exceed 4 ounces/meal) is recommended.

For vegetarians, an increased intake of lima beans and soy products is recommended. Certain spices and herbs such as turmeric, cinnamon, garlic, and ginger can be added to the preparation of vegetables or meat. These spices and herbs have exhibited antioxidant and anti-inflammatory activities. However, it should be remembered that herbal antioxidants as well as standard dietary and endogenous antioxidants produce biological effects (such as changes in gene expression that can produce beneficial effects in patients with diabetes), which may not be related to decreasing oxidative stress or chronic inflammation.

Lifestyle

Lifestyle recommendations include the maintenance of a normal body weight, increasing one's level of physical activity, the cessation of tobacco smoking, stress reduction practices (taking up yoga and/or meditation for instance, and perhaps taking more frequent vacations), and performing moderate exercise. Moderate exercise includes walking twenty to twenty-five minutes a day at least five days a week or using a treadmill (twenty-five minutes at a moderate speed), and weight-lifting for thirty minutes three or four times a week. Given that younger persons can typically do more strenuous exercise than older ones, the level of exercise depends upon the age of the individual.

Primary Prevention Strategies for Type 2 Diabetes

Micronutrient Supplementation

For the primary prevention of type 2 diabetes, an appropriate preparation of multiple-micronutrients is important. Micronutrients include dietary antioxidants (vitamin A, beta-carotene, vitamin C, vitamin E, and selenium) and endogenous antioxidants (alpha-lipoic acid, the glutathione-elevating agent n-acetylcysteine, coenzyme Q10, and L-carnitine), B vitamins, vitamin D, chromium, and the appropriate minerals. The doses of each of these ingredients in a micronutrient formulation differ depending upon the age of the individual. Micronutrient formulations for various age groups having type 1 diabetes (ages five to ten, eleven to seventeen, eighteen to thirty-five, and thirty-six and older) are presented in tables 8.2–8.4. Micronutrient formulations for adults who are obese or who are pre-diabetic (table

8.5) and for patients with diabetic complications (table 8.6) are also provided.

These proposed micronutrient formulations have unique properties that are not found in other multivitamin preparations currently on the market. Full and comprehensive clinical studies on the efficacy of these multiple micronutrients are suggested.

TABLE 8.2. FORMULATION FOR CHILDREN (AGE FIVE TO TEN) WITH TYPE 1 DIABETES*

Vitamin A (palmitate)	1,500 IU
Natural mixed carotenoids	5 mg
Vitamin C (as calcium ascorbate)	100 mg
Vitamin D$_3$ (cholecalciferol)	400 IU
Vitamin E (two forms)	50 IU d-alpha-tocopheryl acetate 25 IU d-alpha-tocopheryl acid succinate 25 IU
Vitamin B$_1$ (thiamine mononitrate)	2 mg
Vitamin B$_2$ (riboflavin)	2 mg
Niacin (as niacinamide ascorbate)	10 mg
Vitamin B$_6$ (pyridoxine HCl)	2 mg
Folate (folic acid)	400 mcg
Vitamin B$_{12}$ (as cyanocobalamin)	5 mcg
Biotin	100 mcg
Pantothenic acid (as d-calcium pantothenate)	5 mg
Calcium citrate	100 mg
Magnesium citrate	50 mg
Zinc glycinate	7.5 mg
Selenium (L-selenomethionine)	50 mcg
Chromium (as chromium picolinate)	25 mcg

*Total capsules per day can be taken orally, half in the morning and half in the evening.

TABLE 8.3. FORMULATION FOR
ADOLESCENTS (AGE 11–17) WITH TYPE 1 DIABETES*

Vitamin A (palmitate)	2,000 IU
Natural mixed carotenoids	5 mg
Vitamin C (as calcium ascorbate)	250 mg
Vitamin D$_3$ (cholecalciferol)	400 IU
Vitamin E (two forms)	100 IU d-alpha-tocopherol acetate 50 IU d-alpha-tocopheryl acid succinate 50 IU
Vitamin B$_1$ (thiamine mononitrate)	2 mg
Vitamin B$_2$ (riboflavin)	2.5 mg
Vitamin B$_3$ (as niacinamide ascorbate)	15 mg
Vitamin B$_6$ (pyridoxine HCl)	2.5 mg
Folate (folic acid)	400 mcg
Vitamin B$_{12}$ (as cyanocobalamin)	10 mcg
Biotin	100 mcg
Pantothenic acid (as d-calcium pantothenate)	5 mg
Calcium citrate	125 mg
Magnesium citrate	62.5 mg
Zinc glycinate	7.5 mg
Selenium (L-selenomethionine)	50 mcg
Chromium (as chromium picolinate)	25 mcg

*Total capsules per day can be taken orally, half in the morning and half in the evening.

TABLE 8.4. FORMULATION FOR
ADULTS (AGE 36+) WITH TYPE 1 OR TYPE 2 DIABETES*

Vitamin A (palmitate)	3,000 IU
Vitamin E (two forms)	400 IU d-alpha-tocopheryl succinate 300 IU d-alpha-tocopheryl acetate 100 IU
Vitamin C (calcium ascorbate)	1,000 mg
Vitamin D$_3$ (cholecalciferol)	800 IU
Vitamin B$_1$ (thiamine mononitrate)	4 mg
Vitamin B$_2$ (riboflavin)	5 mg
Vitamin B$_3$ (niacinamide ascorbate)	30 mg
Vitamin B$_6$ (pyridoxine hydrochloride)	5 mg
Folic acid	800 mcg
Vitamin B$_{12}$ (cyanocobalamin)	10 mcg
Biotin	200 mcg
Pantothenic acid (D-calcium pantothenate)	10 mg
Calcium citrate	250 mg
Magnesium citrate	125 mg
Zinc glycinate	15 mg
Selenium (seleno-L-methionine)	100 mcg
Chromium (as chromium picolinate)	50 mcg
N-acetylcysteine (NAC)	proprietary amount[†]
Coenzyme Q10	proprietary amount
Alpha-lipoic acid	proprietary amount
L-carnitine	proprietary amount
Omega-3 fatty acids	proprietary amount
Natural mixed carotenoids	proprietary amount

*Total capsules per day can be taken orally, half in the morning and half in the evening.
†Total amounts of antioxidants and herbal products come to 865 mg.

PROPOSED RECOMMENDATIONS
FOR SECONDARY PREVENTION

The purpose of secondary prevention, as we have determined, is to stop or slow the progression of diabetes in high-risk populations. Let's look at some secondary prevention strategies for type 1 diabetes next.

Secondary Prevention
Strategies for Type 1 Diabetes

As we know, individuals with a family history (genetic basis) of diabetes develop type 1 diabetes within a few years of birth due to the loss of insulin-producing beta-cells from the pancreas. Therefore, these patients take insulin as soon as a diagnosis is established. Secondary prevention is recommended for patients with type 1 diabetes who are taking insulin but no other glucose-lowering medications.

Micronutrient Supplementation

The formulations for children, adolescents, and adults with type 1 diabetes are described in tables 8.1–8.4. The efficacy of these formulations in individuals who have a family history or who actually have type 1 diabetes should be clinically tested. As well, the proposed strategies for primary and secondary prevention in type 1 and type 2 diabetes patients should be adopted in consultation with a physician.

**The Potential of Multiple-micronutrient
Supplementation in the Prevention of Type 1 Diabetes:
Findings Concerning the Genetic Basis
of Another Disease**

It is often believed that the genetic basis of diabetes cannot be prevented or delayed. However, recent laboratory experiments on the genetic basis of another disease model (cancer) show that it may be possible to prevent or at least delay the onset of the genetic basis of diabetes.

The gene HOP (TUM-1) is essential for the development of *Drosophila melanogaster* (fruit flies). A mutation in this gene markedly increases the risk of developing a leukemia-like tumor in female flies (author's unpublished observation in collaboration with Dr. Bhattacharya et al. of NASA, Moffat Field, California). Proton radiation is a powerful cancer-causing agent. Whole-body irradiation of these flies with proton radiation dramatically increased the incidence of cancer compared to unirradiated flies.

The question arose as to whether or not multiple antioxidants can influence the incidence of cancer, which has a specific gene defect. To test this possibility, a mixture of multiple dietary and endogenous antioxidants was fed to these flies through diet seven days before proton irradiation, and continued throughout the experimental period. The results showed that antioxidant treatment before and after irradiation totally blocked the proton radiation-induced cancer in fruit flies.

This finding on fruit flies is of particular interest because, to my knowledge, this is the first demonstration in which the genetic basis of a disease can be prevented by antioxidant treatment. It is not known whether daily supplementation with antioxidants in women of reproductive age before conception and during their entire pregnancy can prevent or delay the onset of type 1 diabetes in their children. It is also unknown whether daily supplementation with antioxidants soon after birth could prevent or delay the onset of type 1 diabetes. However, the results on fruit flies suggest that daily supplementation with multiple antioxidants could potentially prevent or delay the onset of diabetes in this way.

Secondary Prevention Strategies for Type 2 Diabetes

Secondary prevention is recommended for those individuals with type 2 diabetes who are obese and/or pre-diabetic.

Micronutrient Supplementation

An appropriate preparation of micronutrients containing multiple dietary and endogenous antioxidants is important for the secondary prevention of type 2 diabetes, but they are not currently recommended by state or national agencies. The proposed micronutrient formulation (table 8.5 below) is a new formulation based on the original formulation of Sevak developed by me for Scientific Nutrition and is recommended for those who are obese and/or pre-diabetic. Certain herbs are included because of their beneficial effects in regulating blood levels of glucose. The efficacy of proposed micronutrients formulations should be clinically tested.

TABLE 8.5. FORMULATION FOR
ADULTS WHO ARE OBESE AND/OR PRE-DIABETIC*

Vitamin A (palmitate)	3,000 IU
Vitamin E (two forms)	400 IU d-alpha-tocopheryl succinate 300 IU d-alpha-tocopheryl acetate 100 IU
Vitamin C (calcium ascorbate)	1,000 mg
Vitamin D_3 (cholecalciferol)	800 IU
Vitamin B_1 (thiamine nononitrate)	4 mg
Vitamin B_2 (riboflavin)	5 mg
Vitamin B_3 (niacinamide ascorbate)	30 mg
Vitamin B_6 (pyridoxine hydrochloride)	5 mg
Folic acid	800 mcg
Vitamin B_{12} (cyanocobalamIn)	10 mcg
Biotin	200 mcg
Pantothenic acid (D-calcium antothenate)	10 mg
Calcium citrate	250 mg
Magnesium citrate	125 mg
Zinc glycinate	15 mg

*Total capsules per day can be taken orally, half in the morning and half in the evening.

Selenium (seleno-L-methionine)	100 mcg
Chromium (as chromium picolinate)	100 mcg
N-acetylcysteine (NAC)	proprietary amount[†]
Coenzyme Q10	proprietary amount
Alpha-lipoic acid	proprietary amount
L-carnitine	proprietary amount
Omega-3 fatty acids	proprietary amount
Natural mixed carotenoids	proprietary amount
Cinnamon bark	proprietary amount
Curcumin	proprietary amount
Milk thistle	proprietary amount

†Total amounts of antioxidants and herbal products listed is 1,065 mg.

Changes in Diet and Lifestyle

Dietary and lifestyle changes are also important for the secondary prevention of type 2 diabetes. Recommendations for changes in diet and lifestyle for secondary prevention are the same as those discussed earlier for primary prevention.

Low-dose Aspirin

Although low-dose aspirin (acetylsalicylic acid) at a dose of 81 milligrams per day is commonly recommended for reducing the risk and progression of heart disease, it has shown to be of some value in reducing the risk of diabetes also. As we know, some patients develop aspirin resistance. Although the mechanisms of aspirin-resistance are not known, I suggest that the addition of multiple antioxidants may enhance the effectiveness of low-dose aspirin in reducing platelet aggregation.

This is substantiated by the fact that vitamin E in combination with aspirin is more effective in inhibiting cyclooxygenase-1 (COX-1) enzyme activity than the individual agents (Abate 2000). Thus, supplementation with a preparation of vitamins containing multiple dietary and endogenous antioxidants can prolong the effectiveness of aspirin among semi-responders (those who show a reduced response to aspirin with respect to platelet aggregation) as well as in patients who develop total resistance to aspirin. This should be tested in a well-designed clinical study.

PROPOSED RECOMMENDATIONS
IN COMBINATION WITH STANDARD CARE

Diabetic patients with established type 1 or type 2 diabetes with or without diabetes-related complications and who are undergoing standard care (defined below) are considered suitable candidates for studying the role that antioxidants, together with diet and lifestyle changes, can play in the prevention and management of this disease. As stated previously, no studies have been performed to evaluate the efficacy of a micronutrient preparation containing *multiple* dietary and endogenous antioxidants, B vitamins, vitamin D, chromium picolinate, omega-3 fatty acids, and certain minerals in combination with standard care in the management of diabetes. However, it is the case that such a study has recently been initiated at the Walter Reed National Army Medical Center in Bethesda, Maryland. The results of this study should be available in 2015.

Standard Care with
Anti-diabetic Medications

Standard care of diabetes typically involves the administration of several classes of anti-diabetic drugs that control plasma glucose levels. Standard care with drugs is usually implemented at the doctor's office or in the hospital. Some of the drugs used include the following:

1. **Insulin and long-acting insulin analogues:** These forms of insulin help with glucose uptake and the utilization of glucose in order to maintain normal glucose levels. The long-acting insulin analogues include glargine and detemir.

2. **Drugs stimulating the release of insulin:** These drugs include sulfonylureas, meglitinides, and **repaglinide;** they help to increase the release of insulin from the pancreas.

3. **Drugs improving insulin action:** These drugs include metformin and thiazolidinedione.

4. **Drugs reducing hepatic glucose formation:** This class of drug includes biguanides.

5. **Drugs delaying the digestion and absorption of intestinal carbohydrates:** Carbohydrates are converted to glucose; therefore, reduced absorption may prevent excess accumulation of glucose in the plasma. This class of drugs includes alpha-glucosidase inhibitors.

6. **Glucagon-like peptide-1 (GLP-1) receptor agonists:** These drugs include exanatide and liraglutide.

7. **Drugs inhibiting dipeptidyl peptidase-4 (DPP-4):** These drugs include linagliplin, saxagliptin, sitagliptin, and vildagliptin.

8. **Drug inhibiting a sodium-glucose co-transporter type 2 (SGLT-2):** This class of drugs includes dapagliflozin.

The anti-diabetic drugs mentioned above are used individually or in combination of two or more in an effort to maintain normal plasma glucose levels. As stated previously but bears repeating here, none of these anti-diabetic drugs have an effect on increased oxidative stress and chronic inflammation.

Here are two specific examples of how a multiple-micronutrient formula might help to mitigate these deleterious effects of oxidative stress and inflammation. A potential cure for type 1 diabetes involves the transplantation of islet cells containing insulin-producing beta-cells from the pancreas. Because of this, in severe cases of diabetes with recurrent hyperglycemia, islet cell transplant remains an option for treatment. However, inadequate donor tissue and the adverse effects of immunosuppressive drugs needed to prevent rejection of the transplanted tissue limit their usefulness at this time. Even if we succeed in developing beta-cells that do *not* require immunosuppressive drugs, transplanted beta-cells eventually will die. This is due to the fact that increased oxidative stress and chronic inflammation, which continue to exist, may be one of the causes of loss of beta-cells from the pancreas in type 1 diabetes. Supplementation with multiple antioxidants, acting in a therapeutically synergistic fashion, could therefore prevent the loss of transplanted beta-cells and prolong the effectiveness of these transplanted tissues.

In type 2 diabetes, increased oxidative stress and chronic inflammation may cause damage to the actual beta-cells of the pancreas, and thereby decrease the production and release of insulin. Therefore, the use of multiple antioxidants might be an efficacious choice in this case as well.

The Effects of Micronutrients in Combination with Standard Care

A few studies have explored the potential value of adding up to three micronutrients to improve overall therapeutic efficacy in the prevention and management of diabetes. However, it should be noted that these studies were not long-term studies. They are described here.

In a clinical study involving fifty-two patients with type 2 diabetes who were on typical standard care, supplementation with L-carnitine and simvastatin lowered the serum lipoproteins levels more than a similar study utilizing simvastatin treatment alone (Solfrizzi et al. 2006).

In a clinical study involving seventy-four patients with uncomplicated type 2 diabetes and abnormal lipids, who were on typical standard care, an oral supplementation with coenzyme Q10 (100 milligrams/twice a day) and the cholesterol-lowering drug fenofibrate (200 milligrams/day), or both for twelve weeks, showed that coenzyme Q10 improved blood pressure (systolic and diastolic) and long-term glycemic control, whereas fenofibrate improved lipid profiles but it did not alter blood pressure or glycemic control (Hodgson et al. 2002).

Statins decrease the level of coenzyme Q10 that may interfere with the improvement in blood-vessel function. In a clinical study involving twenty-three patients with type 2 diabetes who were receiving statins, and who were on typical standard care, supplementation with coenzyme Q10 improved blood-vessel function (Hamilton et al. 2009).

In a clinical study with forty-eight overweight and obese men with type 2 diabetes who were on metformin (1,500 milligrams/day), it was demonstrated that supplementation with folic acid (5 milligrams/day) for a period of eight weeks reduced levels of fasting blood glucose, serum insulin, insulin resistance, and HbA1c compared to those who received placebo pills instead of folic acid (Gargari et al. 2011).

In a clinical study with 447 patients with poorly controlled type 2 diabetes who were on oral anti-diabetic medications, supplementation with chromium picolinate (600 micrograms/day) and biotin (2 milligrams/day) for a period of ninety days reduced the levels of fasting blood glucose and hemoglobin A1c (HbA1c) compared to those who received the placebo pills (Albarracin et al. 2008). The studies presented in this section suggest that antioxidants, B-vitamin or chromium, tested in combination with standard therapy produce some beneficial effects in patients with diabetes more than that produced by standard therapy alone. According to this author, the use of multiple-micronutrients as proposed here could have produced stronger beneficial effects than those observed with a single agent.

PROPOSED RECOMMENDATIONS IN COMBINATION WITH STANDARD CARE

In order to produce an optimal benefit in reducing the progression of type 1 and type 2 diabetes, I propose a formulation of multiple-micronutrients and changes in diet and lifestyle in combination with standard care.

Micronutrient Supplementation

The micronutrient formulation I would recommend is referred to as Metabolic.* It has been patented (I am senior author of this patent) by the Premier Micronutrient Corporation (PMC) and is currently being marketed to consumers. This formulation is based on the Sevak formulation developed by me for Scientific Nutrition; it is expressed in table 8.6 on page 157. The addition of omega-3 fatty acids derived from plant sources (alpha-linolenic acid or ALA) rather than fish sources was considered essential because of its beneficial effects in reducing some of the risk factors for diabetes.

Changes in Diet and Lifestyle

These recommendations are the same as those described for the primary prevention of diabetes found earlier in this chapter. (Most doctors have no objection to making these recommendations.)

CONCLUDING REMARKS

In this chapter, I have proposed various recommendations for the primary and secondary prevention of diabetes, including for those individuals currently undergoing standard care.

As regards this, it is expected that the addition of a preparation of micronutrients and diet and lifestyle changes to the regimen of standard care may improve the effectiveness of diabetes treatment and may even reduce the potential harmful effects of anti-diabetic drugs. For example, statins that decrease cholesterol levels also inhibit the formation of coenzyme Q10, because this antioxidant is in the same pathway as cholesterol formation. (Coenzyme Q10, as we know, is needed for energy production by the mitochondria.)

---

*The same formulation with an additional supplement of arginine could be taken by patients who have developed microvessel disease, such as wounds that are difficult to heal due to poor blood supply. The addition of arginine, which can produce increased amounts of nitric oxide (NO), is considered important because NO can dilate small blood vessels and improve the blood supply to the wounds, thereby enhancing the healing process. One's doctor can help to determine the specific amount of arginine supplementation that should be taken.

TABLE 8.6. A FORMULATION FOR ADULTS WHO HAVE ESTABLISHED TYPE 1 DIABETES OR TYPE 2 DIABETES WITH COMPLICATIONS*

Vitamin A (palmitate)	3,000 IU
Vitamin E (two forms)	300 IU d-alpha-tocopheryl succinate 200 IU d-alpha-tocopheryl acetate 100 IU
Vitamin C (calcium ascorbate)	1,000 mg
Vitamin D_3 (cholecalciferol)	1,000 IU
Vitamin B_1 (thiamine mononitrate)	2 mg
Vitamin B_2 (riboflavin)	2 mg
Vitamin B_3 (niacinamide ascorbate)	50 mg
Vitamin B_6 (pyridoxine hydrochloride)	10 mg
Folic acid	5 mg
Vitamin B_{12} (cyanocobalamln)	50 mcg
Biotin	400 mcg
Pantothenic acid (D-calcium pantothenate)	15 mg
Zinc glycinate	15 mg
Selenium (seleno-L-methionine)	125 mcg
Chromium (as chromium picolinate)	200 mcg
N-acetylcysteine (NAC)	proprietary dose[†]
Coenzyme Q10	proprietary dose
Alpha-lipoic acid	proprietary dose
L-carnitine	proprietary dose
Omega-3 fatty acids from plants (as alpha-linolenic acid)	proprietary dose
Natural mixed carotenoids	proprietary dose
Cinnamon bark	proprietary dose
Curcumin	proprietary dose
Milk thistle	proprietary dose
Arginine	proprietary dose

*Total capsules per day can be taken orally, half in the morning and half in the evening.

†Total amount of antioxidants and herbal products is 1,875 mg.

Full clinical studies to test the effectiveness of these recommendations should be initiated. In the meantime, those who are suffering from diabetes should consider adopting them in consultation with their doctors.

The Incidence and Prevalence of Diabetes

INCIDENCE

The annual incidence of newly diagnosed cases of diabetes among individuals age eighteen to seventy-nine has increased from 493,000 in 1980 to 1.7 million in 2010, which is more than a threefold increase. It is interesting to note that there was no significant change in the annual incidence of newly diagnosed cases of diabetes between 2008 and 2010 (CDC Diabetes Data and Trends 2012). The extent of increase in the incidence of diabetes was age-dependent (table A1.1 on page 160).

Although the incidence of diabetes in men and women was similar in 1980, the increase in the annual incidence of newly diagnosed cases of diabetes in men and women was slightly different, with the incidence being slightly higher in men. In men, the incidence increased from 3.4 cases per 1,000 individuals in 1980 to 9.7 cases per 1,000 individuals in 2010. In women, it increased from 3.5 new cases per 1,000 individuals to 7.3 cases per 1,000 individuals.

The incidence of newly diagnosed cases of diabetes varies among different ethnic groups. We know that African Americans have the highest annual incidence of diabetes compared to Caucasians or Latinos; however, the extent of increase from 1997–2010 was the lowest in African Americans (table A1.2 on page 160).

TABLE A1.1. EFFECTS OF AGE ON CHANGES IN THE ANNUAL INCIDENCE OF NEWLY DIAGNOSED DIABETES BETWEEN THE YEARS 1980 AND 2010

Year	Age (years)	Incidence of New Cases per 1,000	Increase
1980	18–44	1.7	
2010	18–44	4.4	2.7-fold
1980	45–64	5.2	
2010	45–64	13.5	2.6-fold
1980	65–79	6.9	
2010	65–79	12.4	1.8-fold

Data were summarized from the CDC Data and Trends, 2012.

TABLE A1.2. EFFECTS OF ETHNICITY ON CHANGES IN THE ANNUAL INCIDENCE OF NEWLY DIAGNOSED CASES OF DIABETES FROM 1997–2010

Year	Ethnic Group	Incidence per 1,000 Persons	Increase in Incidence
1997	Caucasians	4.6	
2010	Caucasians	7.7	1.67-fold
1997	African Americans	9.2	
2010	African Americans	13.0	1.41-fold
1997	Latinos	7.4	
2010	Latinos	12.9	1.74-fold

Data were summarized from the CDC Data and Trends, 2012.

PREVALENCE

Prevalence refers to the total number of people with a disease at a particular year. The prevalence of diagnosed and undiagnosed cases of diabetes in the United States in 2010 varies depending upon age and ethnicity (table A1.3). The total number of diagnosed cases of diabetes was about 18.8 million and undiagnosed cases were about 7 million. About 215,000 individuals younger than age twenty had type 1 or type 2 diabetes in the United States in 2010. Also in 2010, the number of pre-diabetic cases among the U.S. population in individuals who were age twenty or older was 79 million.

TABLE A1.3. PREVALENCE OF DIAGNOSED AND UNDIAGNOSED CASES OF DIABETES IN THE U.S. POPULATION IN 2010

Age/Gender/Ethnicity	Total Number	Percentage of All People
Age 20 or older	25.6 million	11.3
Age 65 or older	10.9 million	26.9
Men age 20 or older	13.0 million	11.8
Women age 20 or older	12.6 million	10.8
Non-Latino Caucasians*	15.7 million	10.2
Non-Latino African Americans	4.9 million	18.7

*Non-Latino Caucasians and non-Latino African Americans were age 20 or older.

Data were summarized from the National Diabetes Information Clearinghouse (NDIC), 2012.

Values of Recommended Dietary Allowances (RDA)/ Dietary Reference Intakes (DRI)

Note to the Reader: All of the information contained in this appendix, including the tables, is from my book *Fighting Cancer with Vitamins and Antioxidants: A Guide to Prevention and Treatment*, coauthored with my son K. C. Prasad, M.S., M.D., published by Healing Arts Press in 2011.

■ ■ ■

Sufficient changes in nutritional guidelines have occurred since World War II, in keeping with increased knowledge of nutrition and health. The nutritional guidelines referred to as Recommended Dietary Allowances (RDAs) were first established in 1941. The Food and Nutrition Board of the United States subsequently revises these guidelines every five to ten years.

RDA (DRI)

RDA refers to the value of the daily dietary intake level of a nutrient considered sufficient to meet the requirements of 97 to 98 percent of healthy individuals of different ages and gender. Because of the rapid growth of research on the role of nutrients in human health, the Food and Nutrition Board of the Institute of Medicine (IOM) of the United States, in collaboration with Health Canada, updated the values of RDAs and renamed them Dietary Reference Intakes (DRI) in 1998. Since then, the DRI values have been used by both countries. The DRI values of selected nutrients are listed in tables A2.1 through A2.21. The DRI values are not currently used in nutrition labeling; the RDA values continue to be used for this purpose. The DRI values for carotenoids, alpha-lipoic acid, n-acetylcysteine, coenzyme Q10, and L-carnitine have not been determined.

ADEQUATE INTAKE (AI)

AI refers to the value of a nutrient for which no RDA has been established, but the value established may be sufficient for everyone in the demographic group.

TOLERABLE UPPER INTAKE LEVEL (UL)

This is the maximum level of daily nutrient intake that is likely to pose no risk of adverse health effects. The UL value represents the total intake of a nutrient from food, water, and supplements.

THE RELATIONSHIP BETWEEN OPTIMAL HEALTH AND RDA VALUES

RDA values of nutrients are expected to be adequate for individuals, for normal growth and survival; however, the values of micronutrients needed for the prevention or the improved management of human diseases are not known at this time. The data on doses obtained from the use of a single micronutrient in the prevention or treatment of human diabetes should not be extrapolated to the doses of the same micronutrient when part of a multiple-micronutrient preparation. Generally, whenever a single micronutrient is used in the laboratory to evaluate its growth-inhibitory effect on cancer cells, therapeutic doses that do not affect the growth of normal cells are needed to observe this effect.

In order to evaluate the dosage of micronutrients in any multivitamin preparation for the prevention or improved treatment of diabetes, it is essential to have sufficient knowledge of the RDA values of the micronutrients.

TABLE A2.1. DIETARY REFERENCE INTAKES (DRI) OF ANTIOXIDANT VITAMIN A

Age	RDA/AI*	UL
	µg/d (IU/d)	µg/d (IU/d)
Infants		
0–6 mo	400 (1,200 IU)*	600 (1,800 IU)
7–12 mo	500 (1,500 IU)*	600 (1,800 IU)
Children		
1–3 y	300 (900 IU)	600 (1,800 IU)
4–8 y	400 (1,200 IU)	900 (2,700 IU)
Males		
9–13 y	600 (1,800 IU)	1,700 (5,100 IU)
14–18 y	900 (2,700 IU)	2,800 (8,400 IU)
19 y and up	900 (2,700 IU)	3,000 (9,000 IU)
Females		
9–13 y	600 (1,800 IU)	1,700 (5,100 IU)
14–18 y	700 (2,100 IU)	2,800 (8,400 IU)
19 y and up	700 (2,100 IU)	3,000 (9,000 IU)
Pregnancy		
under 18 y	750 (2,250 IU)	2,800 (8,400 IU)
19–50 y	770 (2310 IU)	3,000 (9,000 IU)
Lactation		
under 18 y	1,200 (3,600 IU)	2,800 (8,400 IU)
19–50 y	1,300 (3,900 IU)	3,000 (9,000 IU)

I µg of retinol equals I µg of RAE (retinol activity equivalent); I IU of retinol equals 0.3 µg of retinol; and 2 µg of beta-carotene equals I µg of retinol.

RDA = Recommended Dietary Allowance
*AI = Adequate Intake
UL = Tolerable Upper Intake Value
µg = microgram; d = day

The values are adapted and summarized from the table of the Dietary Reference Intakes (DRI) published by www.nap.edu. (Search on "Food and Nutrition" and you will find information about DRI.)

TABLE A2.2. DIETARY REFERENCE
INTAKES (DRI) OF ANTIOXIDANT VITAMIN C

Age	RDA/AI*	UL
	mg/d	mg/d
Infants		
0–6 mo	40*	ND
7–12 mo	50*	ND
Children		
1–3 y	15	400
4–8 y	25	650
Males		
9–13 y	45	1,200
14–18 y	75	1, 800
19 y and up	90	2,000
Females		
9–13 y	45	1,200
14–18 y	65	1,800
19 y and up	75	2,000

RDA = Recommended Dietary Allowance
*AI = Adequate Intake
UL = Tolerable Upper Intake Value
µg = microgram; d = day

The values are adapted and summarized from the table of the Dietary Reference Intakes (DRI) published by www.nap.edu.

TABLE A2.3. DIETARY REFERENCE
INTAKES (DRI) OF ANTIOXIDANT VITAMIN E

Age	RDA/AI*	UL
	mg/d (IU/d)	mg/d (IU/d)
Infants		
0–6 mo	4 (6 IU)*	ND
7–12 mo	5 (7.5 IU)*	ND
Children		
1–3 y	6 (9 IU)	200 (30 IU)
4–8 y	7 (10.6 IU)	300 (45 IU)
Males		
9–13 y	11 (16.7 IU)	600 (90 IU)
14–18 y	15 (22.8 IU)	800 (120 IU)
19 y and up	15 (22.8 IU)	1,000 (150 IU)
Females		
9–13 y	11 (16.7 IU)	600 (90 IU)
14–18 y	15 (22.8 IU)	800 (120 IU)
19 y and up	15 (22.8 IU)	1,000 (150 IU)
Pregnancy		
under 18 y	15 (22.8 IU)	800 (120 IU)
19–50 y	15 (22.8 IU)	1,000 (150 IU)
Lactation		
under 18 y	19 (28.9 IU)	800 (120 IU)
19–50 y	19 (28.9 IU)	1,000 (150 IU)

RDA = Recommended Dietary Allowance
*AI = Adequate Intake
UL = Tolerable Upper Intake Value
ND = not determined
mg = milligram; d = day
1 IU of vitamin E equals 0.66 mg of d- and 0.45 mg of
dl-alpha-tocopherol

The values are adapted and summarized from the tables of the Dietary Reference Intakes (DRI)
published by www.nap.edu.

TABLE A2.4. DIETARY REFERENCE
INTAKES (DRI) OF VITAMIN D

Age	RDA/AI*	UL
	µg/d (IU/d)	µg/d (IU/d)
Infants		
0–12 mo	5 (200 IU)*	25 (1,000 IU)
Children		
1–8 y	5 (200 IU)*	50 (2,000 IU)
Males		
9–50 y	5 (200 IU)*	50 (2,000 IU)
50–70 y	10 (400 IU)*	50 (2,000 IU)
over 70 y	15 (600 IU)*	50 (2,000 IU)
Females		
9–50 y	5 (200 IU)*	50 (2,000 IU)
50–70 y	10 (400 IU)*	50 (2,000 IU)
under 70 y	15 (600 IU)*	50 (2,000 IU)
Pregnancy		
18–50 y	5 (200 IU)*	50 (2,000 IU)
Lactation		
18–50 y	5 (200 IU)*	50 (2,000 IU)

RDA = Recommended Dietary Allowance
*AI = Adequate Intake
UL = Tolerable Upper Intake Value
µg = microgram; d = day
1 µg of cholecalciferol equals 40 IU (international unit)
of Vitamin D.

The values are adapted and summarized from the tables of the Dietary Reference Intakes (DRI) published by www.nap.edu.

TABLE A2.5. DIETARY REFERENCE INTAKES (DRI) OF VITAMIN B$_1$ (THIAMINE)

Age	RDA/AI*	UL
	mg/d	mg/d
Infants		
0–6 mo	0.2*	ND
7–12 mo	0.3*	ND
Children		
1–3 y	0.5	ND
4–8 y	0.6	ND
Males		
9–13 y	0.9	ND
14 y and up	1.2	ND
Females		
9–13 y	0.9	ND
14–18 y	1.0	ND
19 y and up	1.1	ND
Pregnancy		
18–50 y	1.4	ND
Lactation		
18–50 y	1.4	ND

RDA = Recommended Dietary Allowance
*AI = Adequate Intake
UL = Tolerable Upper Intake Value
ND = not determined
mg = milligram; d = day

The values are adapted and summarized from the tables of the Dietary Reference Intakes (DRI) published by www.nap.edu.

TABLE A2.6. DIETARY REFERENCE
INTAKES (DRI) OF VITAMIN B$_2$ (RIBOFLAVIN)

Age	RDA/AI*	UL
	mg/d	mg/d
Infants		
0–6 mo	0.3*	ND
7–12 mo	0.4*	ND
Children		
1–3 y	0.5	ND
4–8 y	0.6	ND
Males		
9–13 y	0.9	ND
14 y and up	13	ND
Females		
9–13	0.9	ND
14–18 y	1.0	ND
19 y and up	1.1	ND
Pregnancy		
18–50 y	1.4	ND
Lactation		
18–50 y	1.6	ND

RDA = Recommended Dietary Allowance
*AI = Adequate Intake
UL = Tolerable Upper Intake Value
ND = not determined
mg = milligram; d = day

The values are adapted and summarized from the table of the Dietary Reference Intakes (DRI) published by www.nap.edu.

TABLE A2.7. DIETARY REFERENCE INTAKES (DRI) OF VITAMIN B₆

Age	RDA/AI*	UL
	mg/d	mg/d
Infants		
0–6 mo	0.1*	ND
7–12 mo	0.3*	ND
Children		
1–3 y	0.5	30
4–8 y	0.6	40
Males		
9–13 y	1.0	60
14–50 y	1.3	80
50–70 y and up	1.7	100
Females		
9–13 y	1.0	60
14–18 y	1.2	80
19–30 y	1.3	100
50 y and up	1.5	100
Pregnancy		
under 18 y	1.9	80
19–50 y	1.9	100
Lactation		
under 18 y	2.0	80
19–50 y	2.0	100

RDA = Recommended Dietary Allowance
*AI = Adequate Intake
UL = Tolerable Upper Intake Value
ND = not determined
mg = milligram; d = day

The values are adapted and summarized from the table of the Dietary Reference Intakes (DRI) published by www.nap.edu.

TABLE A2.8. DIETARY REFERENCE
INTAKES (DRI) OF VITAMIN B₁₂ (COBALAMIN)

Age	RDA/AI*	UL
	µg/d	µg/d
Infants		
0–6 mo	0.4*	ND
7–12 mo	0.5*	ND
Children		
1–3 y	0.9	ND
4–8 y	1.2	ND
Males		
9–13 y	1.08	ND
14 y and up	2.4	ND
Females		
9–13 y	1.8	ND
14 y and up	2.4	ND
Pregnancy		
18–50 y	2.6	ND
Lactation		
18–50 y	2.8	ND

RDA = Recommended Dietary Allowance
*AI = Adequate Intake
UL = Tolerable Upper Intake Value
ND = not determined
µg = microgram; d = day

The values are adapted and summarized from the table of the Dietary Reference Intakes (DRI) published by www.nap.edu.

TABLE A2.9. DIETARY REFERENCE
INTAKES (DRI) OF VITAMIN PANTOTHENIC ACID

Age	RDA/AI*	UL
	mg/d	mg/d
Infants		
0–6 mo	1.7*	ND
7–12 mo	1.8*	ND
Children		
1–3 y	2*	ND
4–8 y	2*	ND
Males		
9–13 y	4*	ND
14 y and up	5*	ND
Females		
9–13 y	4*	ND
14 y and up	5*	ND
Pregnancy		
18–50 y	6*	ND
Lactation		
18–50 y	7*	ND

RDA = Recommended Dietary Allowance
*AI = Adequate Intake
UL = Tolerable Upper Intake Value
ND = not determined
mg = milligram; d = day

The values are adapted and summarized from the table of the Dietary Reference Intakes (DRI) published by www.nap.edu.

TABLE A2.10. DIETARY REFERENCE
INTAKES (DRI) OF VITAMIN NIACIN

Age	RDA/AI*	UL
	mg/d	mg/d
Infants		
0–6 mo	2*	ND
7–12 mo	0.4*	ND
Children		
1–3 y	6.0	10
4–8 y	8.0	15
Males		
9–13 y	12	20
14–50 y	16	30
50 y and up	16	35
Females		
9–13 y	12	20
14–18 y	14	30
19 y and up	14	35
Pregnancy		
under 18 y	18	30
19–50 y	18	35
Lactation		
under 18 y	17	30
19–50 y	17	35

RDA = Recommended Dietary Allowance
*AI = Adequate Intake
UL = Tolerable Upper Intake Value
ND = not determined
mg = milligram; d = day

The values are adapted and summarized from the table of the Dietary Reference Intakes (DRI) published by www.nap.edu

TABLE A2.11. DIETARY REFERENCE INTAKES (DRI) OF VITAMIN FOLATE

Age	RDA/AI*	UL
	µg/d	µg/d
Infants		
0–6 mo	65*	ND
7–12 mo	80*	ND
Children		
1–3 y	150	300
4–8 y	200	400
Males		
9–13 y	300	600
14–18 y	400	800
19 y and up	400	1,000
Females		
9–13 y	300	600
14–18 y	400	800
19 y and up	400	1,000
Pregnancy		
under 18 y	600	800
19–50 y	600	1,000
Lactation		
under 18 y	500	800
19–50 y	500	1,000

RDA = Recommended Dietary Allowance
*AI = Adequate Intake
UL = Tolerable Upper Intake Value
ND = not determined
µg = microgram; d = day

The values are adapted and summarized from the table of the Dietary Reference Intakes (DRI) published by www.nap.edu.

TABLE A2.12. DIETARY REFERENCE
INTAKES (DRI) OF MICRONUTRIENT BIOTIN

Age	RDA/AI*	UL
	µg/d	µg/d
Infants		
0–6 mo	0.5*	ND
7–12 mo	0.6*	ND
Children		
1–3 y	8*	ND
4–8 y	12*	ND
Males		
9–13 y	20	ND
14–18 y	25	ND
19 y and up	30	ND
Females		
9–13 y	20	ND
14–18 y	25	ND
19 y and up	30	ND
Pregnancy		
under 18 y	30*	ND
19–50 y	30*	ND
Lactation		
under 18 y	35*	ND
19–50 y	35*	ND

RDA = Recommended Dietary Allowance
*AI = Adequate Intake
UL = Tolerable Upper Intake Value
ND = not determined
µg = microgram; d = day

The values are adapted and summarized from the table of the Dietary Reference Intakes (DRI) published by www.nap.edu.

TABLE A2.13. DIETARY REFERENCE INTAKES (DRI) OF MINERAL CALCIUM

Age	RDA/AI*	UL
	mg/d	mg/d
Infants		
0–6 mo	210*	ND
7–12 mo	270*	ND
Children		
1–3 y	500*	2,500
4–8 y	800*	2,500
Males		
9–18 y	1,300*	2,500
19–50 y	1,000*	2,500
51 y and up	1,200*	2,500
Females		
9–8 y	1,300*	2,500
19–50 y	1,000*	2,500
51 y and up	1,200*	2,500
Pregnancy		
under 18 y	1,300*	2,500
19–50 y	1,000*	2,500
Lactation		
under 18 y	1,300*	2,500
19–50 y	1,000*	2,500

RDA = Recommended Dietary Allowance
*AI = Adequate Intake
UL = Tolerable Upper Intake Value
ND = not determined
mg = milligram; d = day

The values are adapted and summarized from the table of the Dietary Reference Intakes (DRI) published by www.nap.edu.

TABLE A2.14. DIETARY REFERENCE INTAKES (DRI) OF MINERAL MAGNESIUM

Age	RDA/AI*	UL
	mg/d	mg/d
Infants		
0–6 mo	30*	ND
7–12 mo	75*	ND
Children		
1–3 y	80	65
4–8 y	130	110
Males		
9–13 y	240	350
14–18 y	410	350
19–30 y	400	350
31 y and up	420	350
Females		
9–13 y	240	350
14–18 y	360	350
31 y and up	320	350
Pregnancy		
under 18 y	400	350
19–30 y	350	350
31–50 y	360	350
Lactation		
under 18 y	360	350
31–50 y	320	350

RDA = Recommended Dietary Allowance
*AI = Adequate Intake
UL = Tolerable Upper Intake Value
ND = not determined
mg = milligram; d = day

The values are adapted and summarized from the table of the Dietary Reference Intakes (DRI) published by www.nap.edu.

TABLE A2.15. DIETARY REFERENCE INTAKES (DRI) OF MINERAL MANGANESE

Age	RDA/AI*	UL
	mg/d	mg/d
Infants		
0–6 mo	0.003*	ND
7–12 mo	0.6*	ND
Children		
1–3 y	1.2 *	2
4–8 y	1.5*	3
Males		
9–13 y	1.9*	6
14–18 y	2.2*	9
19 y and up	2.3*	11
Females		
9–13 y	1.6*	6
14–18 y	1.6 *	9
19 y and up	1.8*	11
Pregnancy		
under 18 y	2.0*	9
19–50 y	2.0*	11
Lactation		
under 18 y	2.6*	9
19–50 y	2.6*	11

RDA = Recommended Dietary Allowance
*AI = Adequate Intake
UL = Tolerable Upper Intake Value
ND = not determined
mg = milligram; d = day

The values are adapted and summarized from the table of the Dietary Reference Intakes (DRI) published by www.nap.edu.

TABLE A2.16. DIETARY REFERENCE
INTAKES (DRI) OF MINERAL CHROMIUM

Age	RDA/AI*	UL
	µg/d	µg/d
Infants		
0–6 mo	0.2*	ND
7–12 mo	5.5*	ND
Children		
1–3 y	11*	ND
4–8 y	15*	ND
Males		
9–13 y	25*	ND
14–50 y	35*	ND
51 y and up	30*	ND
Females		
9–13 y	21*	ND
14–18 y	24*	ND
19–50 y	25*	ND
Pregnancy		
under 18 y	29*	ND
19–50 y	30*	ND
Lactation		
under 18 y	44*	ND
19–50 y	45*	ND

RDA = Recommended Dietary Allowance
*AI = Adequate Intake
UL = Tolerable Upper Intake Value
ND = not determined
µg = microgram; d = day

The values are adapted and summarized from the table of the Dietary Reference Intakes (DRI)
published by www.nap.edu.

TABLE A2.17. DIETARY REFERENCE INTAKES (DRI) OF MINERAL COPPER

Age	RDA/AI*	UL
	µg/d	µg/d
Infants		
0–6 mo	200*	ND
7–12 mo	220*	ND
Children		
1–3 y	340	1,000
4–8 y	440	3,000
Males		
9–13 y	700	5,000
14–18 y	890	8,000
19 y and up	900	10,000
Females		
9–13 y	700	5,000
14–18 y	890	8,000
19 y and up	900	10,000
Pregnancy		
under 18 y	1,000	8,000
19–50 y	1,000	10,000
Lactation		
under 18 y	1,300	8,000
19–50 y	1,300	10,000

RDA = Recommended Dietary Allowance
*AI = Adequate Intake
UL = Tolerable Upper Intake Value
ND = not determined
µg = microgram; d = day

The values are adapted and summarized from the table of the Dietary Reference Intakes (DRI) published by www.nap.edu.

TABLE A2.18. DIETARY REFERENCE
INTAKES (DRI) OF MINERAL IRON

Age	RDA/AI*	UL
	mg/d	mg/d
Infants		
0–6 mo	0.27*	40
7–12 mo	11	40
Children		
1–3 y	7	40
4–8 y	10	40
Males		
9–13 y	8	40
14–18 y	11	45
19 y and up	8	45
Females		
9–13 y	8	40
14–18 y	15	45
19–50 y	18	45
50 y and up	8	45
Pregnancy		
18–50 y	27	45
Lactation		
under 18 y	10	45
19–50 y	9	45

RDA = Recommended Dietary Allowance
*AI = Adequate Intake
UL = Tolerable Upper Intake Value
ND = not determined
mg = milligram; d = day

The values are adapted and summarized from the table of the Dietary Reference Intakes (DRI) published by www.nap.edu.

TABLE A2.19. DIETARY REFERENCE INTAKES (DRI) OF MINERAL SELENIUM

Age	RDA/AI*	UL
	µg/d	µg/d
Infants		
0–6 mo	15*	45
7–12 mo	20*	60
Children		
1–3 y	20	90
4–8 y	30	150
Males		
9–13 y	40	280
14 y and up	55	400
Females		
9–13 y	40	280
14 y and up	55	400
Pregnancy		
18–50 y	60	400
Lactation		
18–50 y	70	400

RDA = Recommended Dietary Allowance
*AI = Adequate Intake
UL = Tolerable Upper Intake Value
ND = not determined
µg = microgram; d = day

The values are adapted and summarized from the table of the Dietary Reference Intakes (DRI) published by www.nap.edu.

TABLE A2.20. DIETARY REFERENCE
INTAKES (DRI) OF MINERAL PHOSPHORUS

Age	RDA/AI*	UL
	mg/d	mg/d
Infants		
0–6 mo	100*	ND
7–12 mo	275*	ND
Children		
1–3 y	460	3,000
4–8 y	500	3,000
Males		
9–18 y	1,250	4,000
19–70 y	700	4,000
70 y and up	700	3,000
Females		
9–18 y	1,250	4,000
19–70 y	700	4,000
70 y and up	700	3,000
Pregnancy		
under 18 y	1,250	3,500
19–50 y	700	3,500
Lactation		
under 18 y	1,250	4,000
19–50 y	700	4,000

RDA = Recommended Dietary Allowance
*AI = Adequate Intake
UL = Tolerable Upper Intake Value
ND = not determined
mg = milligram; d = day

The values are adapted and summarized from the table of the Dietary Reference Intakes (DRI) published by www.nap.edu.

TABLE A2.21. DIETARY REFERENCE INTAKES (DRI) OF MINERAL ZINC

Age	RDA/AI*	UL
	mg/d	mg/d
Infants		
0–6	2*	4
7–12 mo	3	5
Children		
1–3 y	3	7
4–8 y	5	12
Males		
9–13 y	8	23
14–18 y	11	34
19 y and up	11	40
Females		
9–13 y	8	23
14–18 y	9	34
19 y and up	8	40
Pregnancy		
under 18 y	12	34
19–50 y	11	40
Lactation		
under 18 y	13	34
19–50 y	12	40

RDA = Recommended Dietary Allowance
*AI = Adequate Intake
UL = Tolerable Upper Intake Value
ND = not determined
mg = milligram; d = day

The values are adapted and summarized from the table of the Dietary Reference Intakes (DRI) published by www.nap.edu.

TABLE A2.22. CALORIE CONTENT
OF SELECTED FOODS

Food	Portion Size	Calories
Apple	1	80
Banana	1	100
Beans, green cooked	½ cup	18
Bread, whole wheat	1 slice	56
Butter	1 tablespoon	100
Carrot	1 medium	34
Cheese	1 ounce	107–14
Corn on the cob	5½ inches	160
Egg	1 large	80
Ice cream	½ cup	135
Kidney beans, cooked	½ cup	110
Meat	3 ounces	200–250
Milk, whole	1 cup	150
Milk, skim	1 cup	85
Orange	1	65
Peach	1	38
Peanuts	1 ounce	172
Pear	1	100
Peas	½ cup	86
Potato chips	10 chips	115
Rice, cooked	½ cup	10
Shrimp	3 ounces	78
Tuna	3 ounces	78
Yogurt, low fat	1 cup	140

From K. N. Prasad and K. C. Prasad, *Fight Cancer with Vitamins and Supplements: A Guide to Prevention and Treatment*, Rochester, Vt.: Healing Arts Press, 2001.

TABLE A2.23. FAT CONTENT
OF SELECTED FOODS

Food	Portion Size	Grams/Portion
Avocado	$1/_8$	4
Bacon, crisp	2 slices	6
Beef, roast	3 ounces	26
Biscuit	1	4
Bread, whole wheat	1 slice	1
Cheese, cheddar	1 ounce	9
Chicken, baked, with skin	3 ounces	11
Chicken, baked, without skin	3 ounces	6
Cornbread	1 piece	7
Egg, boiled	1	6
Ice cream	½ cup	7
Margarine	1 teaspoon	4
Mayonnaise	1 tablespoon	11
Milk, whole	1 cup	8
Milk, skim	1 cup	1
Oatmeal, cooked	½ cup	1
Peanut butter	1 tablespoon	7
Pork chop	3 ounces	19
Shrimp	3 ounces	0.9
Sour cream	1 tablespoon	3
Tuna	3 ounces	0.9
Vegetable oil	1 teaspoon	5
Yogurt, low fat	1 cup	4

From K. N. Prasad and K. C. Prasad, *Fight Cancer with Vitamins and Supplements: A Guide to Prevention and Treatment*, Rochester, Vt.: Healing Arts Press, 2001.

TABLE A2.24. FIBER CONTENT
OF SELECTED FOODS

Food	Portion Size	Grams/Portion
Apple, with skin	1	3
Bread, white	1 slice	0.8
Bread, whole wheat	1 slice	1.3
Broccoli	½ cup	3.2
Carrot, raw	1 medium	2.4
Cereal, all-bran	1 cup	25.6
Cereal, raisin bran	1 cup	6
Corn	½ cup	4.6
Muffin, bran	1	4.2
Pear, with skin	1	3.8
Raspberries	½ cup	4.6

From K. N. Prasad and K. C. Prasad, *Fight Cancer with Vitamins and Supplements: A Guide to Prevention and Treatment*, Rochester, Vt.: Healing Arts Press, 2001.

CONCLUDING REMARKS

The initial nutritional guidelines, Recommended Dietary Allowances (RDAs), have been replaced by Dietary Reference Intakes (DRIs) and are currently used by the United States and Canada. The DRI values of nutrients are sufficient for the growth and development of the 97 to 98 percent of healthy individuals. The DRI values for carotenoids, alpha-lipoic acid, n-acetylcysteine, coenzyme Q10, and L-carnitine have not been determined.

Abbreviations and Terminologies

AA: Arachidonic acid

AEG: Advanced glycation end-products, a marker of diabetes

ALA: Alpha-linolenic acid, an omega-3 fatty acid derived from plants

CRP: C-reactive protein

DHA: Docosahexaenoic acid, a form of omega-3 fatty acid derived from fish

DRI: Dietary Reference Intakes

EPA: Eicosapentaenoic acid, a form of omega-3 fatty acid derived from fish

Extracorpuscular hemoglobin: free hemoglobin in plasma

Glycation: A process during which glucose attaches to proteins or fats without the help of an enzyme

Glycemic index: The value of glucose levels in the plasma

HbA1c: Glycated hemoglobin, a marker of diabetes

Hp: Haptoglobin is an antioxidant protein that protects against oxidative damage

Hyperglycemia: Plasma level of glucose higher than the normal value

Hypertension: High blood pressure

Hypoglycemia: Plasma level of glucose lower than the normal value

IL-6: Interleukin-6, a pro-inflammatory cytokine

Incidence: Annual rate of a disease occurrence

Ischemia: Reduced oxygen

MDA: Malondialdehyde, a marker of oxidative stress

Microalbuminuria: An excess of albumin in the urine, which is an indicator of kidney damage

NAC: N-acetylcysteine

NAD+: Nicotinamide adenine dinucleotide, an oxidizing agent

NADH: The reduced form of NAD+, a reducing agent

Nephropathy: Damage to the kidneys

Neuropathy: Damage to the nerve cells

Nitrosylative damage: Damage produced by free radicals derived from nitrogen

NO: Nitric oxide

NOS: Nitric oxide synthase, an enzyme that makes NO

Oxidation: A process in which an atom or molecule gains oxygen, loses hydrogen, or loses electron

Oxidative damage: Damage produced by free radicals derived from oxygen

Oxidative stress: When production of free radicals surpasses the antioxidant capacity of the body to neutralize them

Periodontics: Gum disease

Prevalence: The total number of people with a disease in a population

Proteinuria: The secretion of an excess of proteins in the urine, a sign of kidney damage

RDA: Recommended Dietary Allowance

Reduction: A process in which an atom or molecule loses oxygen, gains hydrogen, or gains an electron

Retinopathy: Damage to the eyes

ROS: Reactive oxygen species (free radicals derived from oxygen)

SOD: Superoxide dismutase, an antioxidant enzyme made in the body

TNF-alpha: Tumor necrosis factor-alpha, a pro-inflammatory cytokine

Bibliography

Abate, A., G. Yang, P. A. Dennery, et al. 2000. "Synergictic Inhibition of Cyclooxygenase-2 Expression by Vitamin E and Aspirin." *Free Radic Biol* 29: 1135–42.

Aghamohammadi, V., B. P. Gargari, and A. Aliasgharzadeh. 2011. "Effect of Folic Acid Supplementation on Homocysteine, Serum Total Antioxidant Capacity, and Malondialdehyde in Patients with Type 2 Diabetes Mellitus." *Journal of American College of Nutrition* 30, no. 3: 210–15.

Albarracin, C. A., B. C. Fuqua, J. L. Evans, et al. 2008. "Chromium Picolinate and Biotin Combination Improves Glucose Metabolism in Treated, Uncontrolled Overweight to Obese Patients with Type 2 Diabetes." *Diabetes/Metabolism Research and Reviews* 24, no. 1: 41–51.

Ali, A., Y. Ma, J. Reynolds, et al. 2011. "Chromium Effects on Glucose Tolerance and Insulin Sensitivity in Persons at Risk for Diabetes Mellitus." *Endocrine Practice: Official Journal of the American College of Endocrinology and the American Association of Clinical Endocrinologists* 17, no. 1: 16–25.

Alian, Z., M. Hashemipour, E. H. Dehkordi, et al. 2012. "The Effects of Folic Acid on Markers of Endothelial Function in Patients with Type 1 Diabetes Mellitus." *Medicinski Arhiv [Medical Archives]* 66, no. 1: 12–15.

Anderson, R. A., L. M. Evans, G. R. Ellis, et al. 2006. "Prolonged Deterioration of Endothelial Dysfunction in Response to Postprandial Lipaemia Is Attenuated by Vitamin C in Type 2 Diabetes." *Diabetic Medicine* 23, no. 3: 258–64.

Andersson, S. A., A. H. Olsson, J. L. Esguerra, et al. 2012. "Reduced Insulin Secretion Correlates with Decreased Expression of Exocytotic Genes in Pancreatic Islets from Patients with Type 2 Diabetes." *Molecular and Cellular Endocrinology* 364: 36–45.

Appendino, G., G. Belcaro, U. Cornelli, et al. 2011. "Potential Role of Curcumin Phytosome (Meriva) in Controlling the Evolution of Diabetic Microangiopathy, a Pilot Study." *Panminerva Medica* 53, no. 3, suppl 1: 43–49.

Arnlov, J., B. Zethelius, U. Riserus, et al. 2009. "Serum and Dietary Beta-carotene and Alpha-tocopherol and Incidence of Type 2 Diabetes Mellitus in a Community-based Study of Swedish Men: Report from the Uppsala Longitudinal Study of Adult Men (ULSAM) Study." *Diabetologia* 52, no. 1: 97–105.

Aroor, A. R., C. Mandavia, J. Ren, et al. 2012. "Mitochondria and Oxidative Stress in the Cardiorenal Metabolic Syndrome." *Cardiorenal Medicine* 2, no. 2: 87–109.

Aukrust, P., L. Gullestad, K. T. Lappegard, et al. 2001. "Complement Activation in Patients with Congestive Heart Failure: Effect of High-dose Intravenous Immunoglobulin Treatment." *Circulation* 104, no. 13: 1494–1500.

Austin, D. F., D. Konrad-Martin, S. Griest, et al. 2009. "Diabetes-related Changes in Hearing." *The Laryngoscope* 119, no. 9: 1788–96.

Ayaz, M., S. Tuncer, N. Okudan, et al. 2008. "Coenzyme Q(10) and Alpha-lipoic Acid Supplementation in Diabetic Rats: Conduction Velocity Distributions." *Methods and Findings in Experimental Clinical Pharmacology* 30, no. 5: 367–74.

Azar, M., A. Basu, A. J. Jenkins, et al. 2011. "Serum Carotenoids and Fat-soluble Vitamins in Women with Type 1 Diabetes and Preeclampsia: a Longitudinal Study." *Diabetes Care* 34, no. 6: 1258–64.

Badr, G., S. Bashandy, H. Ebaid, et al. 2012. "Vitamin C Supplementation Reconstitutes Polyfunctional T Cells in Streptozotocin-induced Diabetic Rats." *European Journal of Nutrition* 51, no. 5: 623–33.

Bainbridge, K. E., H. J. Hoffman, and C. C. Cowie. 2008. "Diabetes and Hearing Impairment in the United States: Audiometric Evidence from the National Health and Nutrition Examination Survey, 1999 to 2004." *Annals of Internal Medicine* 149, no. 1: 1–10.

Balk, E. M., A. Tatsioni, A. H. Lichtenstein, et al. 2007. "Effect of Chromium Supplementation on Glucose Metabolism and Lipids: a Systematic Review of Randomized Controlled Trials." *Diabetes Care* 30, no. 8: 2154–63.

Bastard, J. P., M. Maachi, C. Lagathu, et al. 2006. "Recent Advances in the Relationship between Obesity, Inflammation, and Insulin Resistance." *European Cytokine Network* 17, no. 1: 4–12.

Bergerhoff, K., C. Clar, and B. Richter. 2002. "Aspirin in Diabetic Retinopathy, a Systematic Review." *Endocrinology Metabolism Clinical North America* 31, no. 3: 779–93.

Berry, D. C., D. DeSantis, H. Soltanian, et al. 2012. "Retinoic Acid Upregulates Preadipocyte Genes to Block Adipogenesis and Suppress Diet-induced Obesity." *Diabetes* 61, no. 5: 1112–21.

Berryman, A. M., A. C. Maritim, R. A. Sanders, et al. 2004. "Influence of Treatment of Diabetic Rats with Combinations of Pycnogenol, Beta-carotene, and Alpha-lipoic Acid on Parameters of Oxidative Stress." *Journal of Biochemistry Molecular Toxicology* 18, no. 6: 345–52.

Bertolotto, F., and A. Massone. 2012. "Combination of Alpha Lipoic Acid and Superoxide Dismutase Leads to Physiological and Symptomatic Improvements in Diabetic Neuropathy." *Drugs in R&D* 12, no. 1: 29–34.

Beydoun, M. A., J. A. Canas, H. A. Beydoun, et al. 2012. "Serum Antioxidant Concentrations and Metabolic Syndrome Are Associated among U.S. Adolescents in Recent National Surveys." *Journal of Nutrition* 142, no. 9: 1693–1704.

Block, K., Y. Gorin, and H. E. Abboud. 2009. "Subcellular Localization of Nox4 and Regulation in Diabetes." *Proceedings of the National Academy of Sciences USA* 106, no. 34: 14385–90.

Boaz, M., L. Lisy, G. Zandman-Goddard, et al. 2009. "The Effect of Anti-inflammatory (Aspirin and/or Statin) Therapy on Body Weight in Type 2 Diabetic Individuals: EAT, a Retrospective Study." *Diabetic Medicine* 26, no. 7: 708–13.

Broadhurst, C. L., and P. Domenico. 2006. "Clinical Studies on Chromium Picolinate Supplementation in Diabetes Mellitus—a Review." *Diabetes Technology Therapy* 8, no. 6: 677–87.

Brostow, D. P., A. O. Odegaard, W. P. Koh, et al. 2011. "Omega-3 Fatty Acids and Incident Type 2 Diabetes: the Singapore Chinese Health Study." *American Journal of Clinical Nutrition* 94, no. 2: 520–26.

Buyukinan, M., S. Ozen, S. Kokkun, et al. 2012. "The Relation of Vitamin D Deficiency with Puberty and Insulin Resistance in Obese Children and Adolescents." *Journal of Pediatric Endocrinology & Metabolism* 25, no. 1–2: 83–87.

Carvalho-Filho, M. A., E. R. Ropelle, R. J. Pauli, et al. 2009. "Aspirin Attenuates Insulin Resistance in Muscle of Diet-induced Obese Rats by Inhibiting

Inducible Nitric Oxide Synthase Production and S-nitrosylation of IRbeta/ IRS-1 and Akt." *Diabetologia* 52: 2425–34.

Cauchi, S., and P. Froguel. 2008. "TCF7L2 Genetic Defect and Type 2 Diabetes." *Current Diabetes Reports* 8, no. 2: 149–55.

Chiu, W. C., Y. C. Hou, C. L. Yeh, et al. 2007. "Effect of Dietary Fish Oil Supplementation on Cellular Adhesion Molecule Expression and Tissue Myeloperoxidase Activity in Diabetic Mice with Sepsis." *British Journal of Nutrition* 97, no. 4: 685–91.

Chui, M. H., and C. E. Greenwood. 2008. "Antioxidant Vitamins Reduce Acute Meal-induced Memory Deficits in Adults with Type 2 Diabetes." *Nutrition Research* 28, no. 7: 423–29.

Cinkilic, N., S. Kiyici, S. Celikler, et al. 2009. "Evaluation of Chromosome Aberrations, Sister Chromatid Exchange and Micronuclei in Patients with Type-1 Diabetes Mellitus." *Mutation Research* 676, no. 1–2: 1–4.

Codoner-Franch, P., S. Pons-Morales, L. Boix-Garcia, et al. 2010. "Oxidant/ Antioxidant Status in Obese Children Compared to Pediatric Patients with Type 1 Diabetes Mellitus." *Pediatric Diabetes* 11: 251–57.

Colwell, J. A. 2004. "Antiplatelet Agents for the Prevention of Cardiovascular Disease in Diabetes Mellitus." *American Journal of Cardiovascular Drugs* 4, no. 2: 87–106.

Cosar, M., A. Songur, and O. Sahin, 2008. "The Neuroprotective Effect of Fish N-3 Fatty Acids in the Hippocampus of Diabetic Rats." *Nutritional Neuroscience* 11, no. 4: 161–66.

Cotran, R. S., V. Kumar, and T. Collins, eds. *Pathologic Basis of Disease*. New York: W. B. Saunders, 1999.

Crawford, J. M., and R. S. Cotran. 1999. "The Pancreas." In *Robbins Pathologic Basis of Disease*. Edited by Cotran, R. S., V. Kumar, and T. Collins. Philadelphia: W.B. Saunders.

Cumurcu, T., D. Mendil, and U. Erkorkmaz. 2008. "Aqueous Humor and Serum Levels of Chromium in Cataract Patients with and without Diabetes Mellitus." *Ophthalmologica Journal International* 222, no. 5: 324–28.

Darmaun, D., S. D. Smith, S. Sweeten, et al. 2008. "Poorly Controlled Type 1 Diabetes Is Associated with Altered Glutathione Homeostasis in Adolescents: Apparent Resistance to N-acetylcysteine Supplementation." *Pediatric Diabetes* 9, no. 6: 577–82.

Davis, P. A., and W. Yokoyama. 2011. "Cinnamon Intake Lowers Fasting Blood

Glucose: Meta-analysis." *Journal of Medicinal Food* 14, no. 9: 884–89.

De Luis, D. A., R. Conde, R. Aller, et al. 2009. "Effect of Omega-3 Fatty Acids on Cardiovascular Risk Factors in Patients with Type 2 Diabetes Mellitus and Hypertriglyceridemia: an Open Study." *European Review of Medical Pharmacological Sciences* 13, no. 1: 51–55.

De Mattia, G., M. C. Bravi, O. Laurenti, et al. 1998. "Reduction of Oxidative Stress by Oral N-acetyl-L-cysteine Treatment Decreases Plasma Soluble Vascular Cell Adhesion Molecule-1 Concentrations in Non-obese, Non-dyslipidaemic, Normotensive, Patients with Non-insulin-dependent Diabetes." *Diabetologia* 41, no. 11: 1392–96.

de Oliveira, A. M., P. H. Rondo, L. A. Luzia, et al. 2011. "The Effects of Lipoic Acid and Alpha-tocopherol Supplementation on the Lipid Profile and Insulin Sensitivity of Patients with Type 2 Diabetes Mellitus: a Randomized, Double-blind, Placebo-controlled Trial." *Diabetes Research and Clinical Practice* 92, no. 2: 253–60.

Djousse, L., M. L. Biggs, R. N. Lemaitre, et al. 2011a. "Plasma Omega-3 Fatty Acids and Incident Diabetes in Older Adults." *American Journal of Clinical Nutrition* 94, no. 2: 527–33.

Djousse, L., J. M. Gaziano, J. E. Buring, et al. 2011b. "Dietary Omega-3 Fatty Acids and Fish Consumption and Risk of Type 2 Diabetes." *American Journal of Clinical Nutrition* 93, no. 1: 143–50.

Donath, M. Y., D. M. Schumann, M. Faulenbach, et al. 2008. "Islet Inflammation in Type 2 Diabetes: from Metabolic Stress to Therapy." *Diabetes Care* 31, suppl 2: S161–64.

Dou, M., A. G. Ma, Q. Z. Wang, et al. 2009. "Supplementation with Magnesium and Vitamin E Was More Effective than Magnesium Alone to Decrease Plasma Lipids and Blood Viscosity in Diabetic Rats." *Nutrition Research* 29, no. 7: 519–24.

Drake, T. C., K. D. Rudser, E. R. Seaquist, et al. 2012. "Chromium Infusion in Hospitalized Patients with Severe Insulin Resistance: a Retrospective Analysis." *Endocrine Practice* 18, no. 3: 394–98.

Ebbesson, S. O., P. M. Risica, L. O. Ebbesson, et al. 2005. "Eskimos Have CHD Despite High Consumption of Omega-3 Fatty Acids: the Alaska Siberia Project." *International Journal of Circumpolar Health* 64, no. 4: 387–95.

Ehses, J. A., G. Lacraz, M. H. Giroix, et al. 2009. "IL-1 Antagonism Reduces Hyperglycemia and Tissue Inflammation in the Type 2 Diabetic GK

Rat." *Proceedings of the National Academy of Sciences USA* 106, no. 33: 13998–14003.

El-ghoroury, E. A., H. M. Raslan, E. A. Badawy, et al. 2009. "Malondialdehyde and Coenzyme Q10 in Platelets and Serum in Type 2 Diabetes Mellitus: Correlation with Glycemic Control." *Blood Coagulation and Fibrinolysis* 20, no. 4: 248–51.

El-Mesallamy, H., N. Hamdy, S. Suwailem, et al. 2010. "Oxidative Stress and Platelet Activation: Markers of Myocardial Infarction in Type 2 Diabetes Mellitus." *Angiology* 61: 14–18.

Erikstrup, C., O. H. Mortensen, A. R. Nielsen, et al. 2009. "RBP-to-retinol Ratio, but Not Total RBP, Is Elevated in Patients with Type 2 Diabetes." *Diabetes, Obesity & Metabolism* 11, no. 3: 204–12.

Ervin, R. B. 2009. "Prevalance of Metabolic Syndrome among Adults 20 Years of Age and Over, by Sex, Age, Race and Ethnicity, and Body Mass Index: United States, 2003–2006." *National Health Statistics Reports* 13.

Evans, J. D., T. F. Jacobs, and E. W. Evans. 2008. "Role of Acetyl-L-carnitine in the Treatment of Diabetic Peripheral Neuropathy." *Annals of Pharmacotherapy* 42, no. 11: 1686–91.

Fraser, D. A., L. M. Diep, I. A. Hovden, et al. 2012. "The Effects of Long-term Oral Benfotiamine Supplementation on Peripheral Nerve Function and Inflammatory Markers in Patients with Type 1 Diabetes: a 24-month, Double-blind, Randomized, Placebo-controlled Trial." *Diabetes Care* 35, no. 5: 1095–97.

Gagnon, C., Z. X. Lu, D. J. Magliano, et al. 2012. "Low Serum 25-hydroxyvitamin D Is Associated with Increased Risk of the Development of the Metabolic Syndrome at Five Years: results from a National, Population-based Prospective Study (The Australian Diabetes, Obesity and Lifestyle Study: AusDiab)." *The Journal of Clinical Endocrinology and Metabolism* 97, no. 6: 1953–61.

Gargari, B. P., V. Aghamohammadi, and A. Aliasgharzadeh. 2011. "Effect of Folic Acid Supplementation on Biochemical Indices in Overweight and Obese Men with Type 2 Diabetes." *Diabetes Research and Clinical Practice* 94, no. 1: 33–38.

Garman, J. H., S. Mulroney, M. Manigrasso, et al. 2009. "Omega-3 Fatty Acid Rich Diet Prevents Diabetic Renal Disease." *American Journal of Physiology and Renal Physiology* 296, no. 2: F306–16.

Gavrilov, V., I. Harman-Boehm, D. Amichay, et al. 2012. "Kidney Function and

Retinol Status in Type 2 Diabetes Mellitus Patients." *Acta Diabetologica* 49, no. 2: 137–43.

Giacco, R., V. Cuomo, B. Vessby, et al. 2007. "Fish Oil, Insulin Sensitivity, Insulin Secretion and Glucose Tolerance in Healthy People: Is There Any Effect of Fish Oil Supplementation in Relation to the Type of Background Diet and Habitual Dietary Intake of N-6 and N-3 Fatty Acids?" *Nutrition Metabolism in Cardiovascular Disease* 17, no. 8: 572–80.

Golias, C., E. Tsoutsi, A. Matziridis, et al. 2007. "Review. Leukocyte and Endothelial Cell Adhesion Molecules in Inflammation Focusing on Inflammatory Heart Disease." *In Vivo* 21, no. 5: 757–69.

Gonzalez-Ortiz, M., E. Martinez-Abundis, J. A. Robles-Cervantes, et al. 2011. "Effect of Thiamine Administration on Metabolic Profile, Cytokines and Inflammatory Markers in Drug-naive Patients with Type 2 Diabetes." *European Journal of Nutrition* 50, no. 2: 145–49.

Gordin, D., C. Forsblom, M. Ronnback, et al. 2008. "Acute Hyperglycaemia Induces an Inflammatory Response in Young Patients with Type 1 Diabetes." *Annals of Medicine* 40, no. 8: 627–33.

Gorin, Y., K. Block, J. Hernandez, et al. 2005. "Nox4 NAD(P)H Oxidase Mediates Hypertrophy and Fibronectin Expression in the Diabetic Kidney." *Journal of Biological Chemistry* 280, no. 47: 39616–26.

Gu, X. M., S. S. Zhang, J. C. Wu, et al. 2010. "[Efficacy and Safety of High-dose Alpha-lipoic Acid in the Treatment of Diabetic Polyneuropathy]." *Zhonghua Yi Xue Za Zhi* 90, no. 35: 2473–76.

Hamblin, M., H. M. Smith, and M. F. Hill. 2007. "Dietary Supplementation with Vitamin E Ameliorates Cardiac Failure in Type I Diabetic Cardiomyopathy by Suppressing Myocardial Generation of 8-iso-prostaglandin F2alpha and Oxidized Glutathione." *Journal of Cardiac Failure* 13, no. 10: 884–92.

Hamden, K., S. Carreau, K. Jamoussi, et al. 2009. "1Alpha,25 Dihydroxyvitamin D3: Therapeutic and Preventive Effects against Oxidative Stress, Hepatic, Pancreatic and Renal Injury in Alloxan-induced Diabetes in Rats." *Journal of Nutritional Science Vitaminology* 55, no. 3: 215–22.

Hamdy, N. M., S. M. Suwailem, and H. O. El-Mesallamy. 2009. "Influence of Vitamin E Supplementation on Endothelial Complications in Type 2 Diabetes Mellitus Patients Who Underwent Coronary Artery Bypass Graft." *Journal of Diabetes Complications* 23, no. 3: 167–73.

Hamilton, S. J., G. T. Chew, and G. F. Watts. 2009. "Coenzyme Q10 Improves

Endothelial Dysfunction in Statin-treated Type 2 Diabetic Patients." *Diabetes Care* 32, no. 5: 810–12.

Harding, A. H., N. J. Wareham, S. A. Bingham, et al. 2008. "Plasma Vitamin C Level, Fruit and Vegetable Consumption, and the Risk of New-onset Type 2 Diabetes Mellitus: the European Prospective Investigation of Cancer—Norfolk Prospective Study." *Archives of Internal Medicine* 168, no. 14: 1493–99.

Haritoglou, C., J. Gerss, H. P. Hammes, et al. 2011. "Alpha-lipoic Acid for the Prevention of Diabetic Macular Edema." *Ophthalmologica Journal International* 226, no. 3: 127–37.

Hartweg, J., A. J. Farmer, R. R. Holman, et al. 2009. "Potential Impact of Omega-3 Treatment on Cardiovascular Disease in Type 2 Diabetes." *Current Opinion in Lipidology* 20, no. 1: 30–38.

Hartweg, J., A. J. Farmer, R. Perera, et al. 2007. "Meta-analysis of the Effects of N-3 Polyunsaturated Fatty Acids on Lipoproteins and Other Emerging Lipid Cardiovascular Risk Markers in Patients with Type 2 Diabetes." *Diabetologia* 50, no. 8: 1593–1602.

Hartweg, J., R. Perera, V. Montori, et al. 2008. "Omega-3 Polyunsaturated Fatty Acids (PUFA) for Type 2 Diabetes Mellitus." *Cochrane Database Systemic Review*, no. 1: CD003205.

Hasanein, P., and S. Shahidi. 2010. "Effects of Combined Treatment with Vitamins C and E on Passive Avoidance Learning and Memory in Diabetic Rats." *Neurobiology of Learning and Memory* 93, no. 4: 472–78.

Hata, I., M. Kaji, S. Hirano, et al. 2006. "Urinary Oxidative Stress Markers in Young Patients with Type 1 Diabetes." *Pediatrics International: Official Journal of the Japan Pediatric Society* 48, no. 1: 58–61.

Hayashino, Y., C. H. Hennekens, and T. Kurth. 2009. "Aspirin Use and Risk of Type 2 Diabetes in Apparently Healthy Men." *American Journal of Medicine* 122, no. 4: 374–79.

Heilbronn, L. K., and L. V. Campbell. 2008. "Adipose Tissue Macrophages, Low Grade Inflammation and Insulin Resistance in Human Obesity." *Current Pharmaceutical Design* 14, no. 12: 1225–30.

Heilman, K., M. Zilmer, K. Zilmer, et al. 2009. "Lower Bone Mineral Density in Children with Type 1 Diabetes Is Associated with Poor Glycemic Control and Higher Serum ICAM-1 and Urinary Isoprostane Levels." *Journal of Bone and Mineral Metabolism* 27, no. 5: 598–604.

Henriksen, E. J. 2006. "Exercise Training and the Antioxidant Alpha-lipoic

Acid in the Treatment of Insulin Resistance and Type 2 Diabetes." *Free Radicals Biology and Medicine* 40, no. 1: 3–12.

Hernandez-Pedro, N., G. Ordonez, A. Ortiz-Plata, et al. 2008. "All-trans Retinoic Acid Induces Nerve Regeneration and Increases Serum and Nerve Contents of Neural Growth Factor in Experimental Diabetic Neuropathy." *Translational Research* 152, no. 1: 31–37.

Hillis, G. S., and A. D. Flapan. 1998. "Cell Adhesion Molecules in Cardiovascular Disease: a Clinical Perspective." *Heart* 79, no. 5: 429–31.

Hino, K., M. Nishikawa, E. Sato, et al. 2005. "L-carnitine Inhibits Hypoglycemia-induced Brain Damage in the Rat." *Brain Research* 1053, no. 1–2: 77–87.

Hodgson, J. M., G. F. Watts, D. A. Playford, et al. 2002. "Coenzyme Q10 Improves Blood Pressure and Glycaemic Control: a Controlled Trial in Subjects with Type 2 Diabetes." *European Journal of Clinical Nutrition* 56, no. 11: 1137–42.

Hoffman, R. P., A. S. Dye, and J. A. Bauer. 2012. "Ascorbic Acid Blocks Hyperglycemic Impairment of Endothelial Function in Adolescents with Type 1 Diabetes." *Pediatric Diabetes* 13: 607–10.

Holvoet, P. 2008. "Relations between Metabolic Syndrome, Oxidative Stress and Inflammation and Cardiovascular Disease." *Verhandelingen—Koninklijke Academie voor Geneeskunde van Belgie* 70, no. 3: 193–219.

House, A. A., M. Eliasziw, D. C. Cattran, et al. 2010. "Effect of B-vitamin Therapy on Progression of Diabetic Nephropathy: a Randomized Controlled Trial." *Journal of American Medical Association* 303, no. 16: 1603–09.

Huang, E. S., A. Basu, M. O'Grady, et al. 2009. "Projecting the Future Diabetes Population Size and Related Costs for the U.S." *Diabetes Care* 32, no. 12: 2225–29.

Huseini, H. F., B. Larijani, R. Heshmat, et al. 2006. "The Efficacy of Silybum Marianum (L.) Gaertn. (Silymarin) in the Treatment of Type II Diabetes: a Randomized, Double-blind, Placebo-controlled, Clinical Trial." *Phytotherapy Research* 20, no. 12: 1036–39.

Hutchinson, M. S., Y. Figenschau, B. Almas, et al. 2011. "Serum 25-hydroxyvitamin D Levels in Subjects with Reduced Glucose Tolerance and Type 2 Diabetes—the Tromso OGTT-study." *International Journal for Vitamin and Nutrition Research* 81, no. 5: 317–27.

Ingold, K. U., G. W. Burton, D. O. Foster, et al. 1987. "Biokinetics of and

Discrimination between Dietary RRR- and SRR-alpha-tocopherols in the Male Rat." *Lipids* 22, no. 3: 163–72.

Iqbal, N., S. Cardillo, S. Volger, et al. 2009. "Chromium Picolinate Does Not Improve Key Features of Metabolic Syndrome in Obese Nondiabetic Adults." *Metabolism Syndrome Related Disorders* 7, no. 2: 143–50.

Jacob, S., P. Ruus, R. Hermann, et al. 1999. "Oral Administration of RAC-alpha-lipoic Acid Modulates Insulin Sensitivity in Patients with Type-2 Diabetes Mellitus: a Placebo-controlled Pilot Trial." *Free Radicals Biology and Medicine* 27, no. 3–4: 309–14.

Jain, S. K., T. Velusamy, J. L. Croad, et al. 2009. "L-cysteine Supplementation Lowers Blood Glucose, Glycated Hemoglobin, CRP, MCP-1, and Oxidative Stress and Inhibits NF-kappaB Activation in the Livers of Zucker Diabetic Rats." *Free Radicals Biology and Medicine* 46, no. 12: 1633–38.

Jariyapongskul, A., T. Rungjaroen, N. Kasetsuwan, et al. 2007. "Long-term Effects of Oral Vitamin C Supplementation on the Endothelial Dysfunction in the Iris Microvessels of Diabetic Rats." *Microvascular Research* 74, no. 1: 32–38.

Jaxa-Chamiec, T., B. Bednarz, K. Herbaczynska-Cedro, et al. 2009. "Effects of Vitamins C and E on the Outcome after Acute Myocardial Infarction in Diabetics: a Retrospective, Hypothesis-generating Analysis from the MIVIT Study." *Cardiology* 112, no. 3: 219–23.

Jialal, I., S. Devaraj, B. Adams-Huet, et al. 2012. "Increased Cellular and Circulating Biomarkers of Oxidative Stress in Nascent Metabolic Syndrome." *The Journal of Clinical Endocrinology and Metabolism* 97: 1844–50.

Jorge, A. G., C. M. Modulo, A. C. Dias, et al. 2009. "Aspirin Prevents Diabetic Oxidative Changes in Rat Lacrimal Gland Structure and Function." *Endocrinology* 35, no. 2: 189–97.

Kabir, M., G. Skurnik, N. Naour, et al. 2007. "Treatment for 2 Mo with N-3 Polyunsaturated Fatty Acids Reduces Adiposity and Some Atherogenic Factors but Does Not Improve Insulin Sensitivity in Women with Type 2 Diabetes: a Randomized Controlled Study." *American Journal of Clinical Nutrition* 86, no. 6: 1670–79.

Kahn, S. E., S. Suvag, L. A. Wright, et al. 2012. "Interactions between Genetic Background, Insulin Resistance and Beta-cell Function." *Diabetes, Obesity & Metabolism* 14, suppl 3: 46–56.

Kajimoto, Y., and H. Kaneto. 2004. "Role of Oxidative Stress in Pancreatic Beta-cell Dysfunction." *Annals of New York Academy of Sciences* 1011: 168–76.

Kamboj, S. S., K. Chopra, and R. Sandhir. 2008. "Neuroprotective Effect of N-acetylcysteine in the Development of Diabetic Encephalopathy in Streptozotocin-induced Diabetes." *Metabolic Brain Disorders* 23, no. 4: 427–43.

Kamboj, S. S., K. Chopra, and R. Sandhir. 2009. "Hyperglycemia-induced Alterations in Synaptosomal Membrane Fluidity and Activity of Membrane Bound Enzymes: Beneficial Effect of N-acetylcysteine Supplementation." *Neuroscience* 162, no. 2: 349–58.

Kataja-Tuomola, M. K., J. P. Kontto, S. Mannisto, et al. 2011. "Intake of Antioxidants and Risk of Type 2 Diabetes in a Cohort of Male Smokers." *European Journal of Clinical Nutrition* 65, no. 5: 590–97.

Kataja-Tuomola, M., J. R. Sundell, S. Mannisto, et al. 2008. "Effect of Alpha-tocopherol and Beta-carotene Supplementation on the Incidence of Type 2 Diabetes." *Diabetologia* 51, no. 1: 47–53.

Kaushik, M., D. Mozaffarian, D. Spiegelman, et al. 2009. "Long-chain Omega-3 Fatty Acids, Fish Intake, and the Risk of Type 2 Diabetes Mellitus." *American Journal of Clinical Nutrition* 90, no. 3: 613–20.

Kennedy, A. R., and N. I. Krinsky. 1994. "Effects of Retinoids, Beta-carotene, and Canthaxanthin on UV- and X-ray-induced Transformation of C3H10T1/2 Cells in Vitro." *Nutrition and Cancer* 22, no. 3: 219–32.

Khajehdehi, P., M. Pakfetrat, K. Javidnia, et al. 2011. "Oral Supplementation of Turmeric Attenuates Proteinuria, Transforming Growth Factor-beta and Interleukin-8 Levels in Patients with Overt Type 2 Diabetic Nephropathy: a Randomized, Double-blind and Placebo-Controlled Study." *Scandinavian Journal of Urology and Nephrology* 45, no. 5: 365–70.

Khan, S., G. V. Raghuram, A. Bhargava, et al. 2011. "Role and Clinical Significance of Lymphocyte Mitochondrial Dysfunction in Type 2 Diabetes Mellitus." *Translational Research: The Journal of Laboratory and Clinical Medicine* 158, no. 6: 344–59.

Kojima, M., L. Sun, I. Hata, et al. 2007. "Efficacy of Alpha-lipoic Acid against Diabetic Cataract in Rat." *Japanese Journal of Ophthalmology* 51, no. 1: 10–13.

Komorowski, J. R., D. Greenberg, and V. Juturu. 2008. "Chromium Picolinate Does Not Produce Chromosome Damage." *Toxicology in Vitro* 22, no. 3: 819–26.

Kostolanska, J., V. Jakus, and L. Barak. 2009. "HbA1c and Serum Levels of Advanced Glycation and Oxidation Protein Products in Poorly and Well Controlled Children and Adolescents with Type 1 Diabetes Mellitus." *Journal of Pediatric Endocrinolology and Metabolism* 22, no. 5: 433–42.

Kotani, K., and N. Sakane. 2012. "C-reactive Protein and Reactive Oxygen Metabolites in Subjects with Metabolic Syndrome." *The Journal of International Medical Research* 40, no. 3: 1074–81.

Kromhout, D., J. M. Geleijnse, J. de Goede, et al. 2011. "N-3 Fatty Acids, Ventricular Arrhythmia-related Events, and Fatal Myocardial Infarction in Postmyocardial Infarction Patients with Diabetes." *Diabetes Care* 34, no. 12: 2515–20.

Kuhad, A., and K. Chopra. 2009. "Attenuation of Diabetic Nephropathy by Tocotrienol: Involvement of NFkB Signaling Pathway." *Life Sciences* 84, no. 9–10: 296–301.

Kumawat, M., T. K. Sharma, N. Singh, et al. 2012. "Study of Changes in Antioxidant Enzymes Status in Diabetic Post Menopausal Group of Women Suffering from Cardiovascular Complications." *Clinical Laboratory* 58, 3–4: 203–07.

Lai, M. H. 2008. "Antioxidant Effects and Insulin Resistance Improvement of Chromium Combined with Vitamin C and E Supplementation for Type 2 Diabetes Mellitus." *Journal of Clinical Biochemistry and Nutrition* 43, no. 3: 191–98.

Lee, C. T., E. L. Gayton, J. W. Beulens, et al. 2010. "Micronutrients and Diabetic Retinopathy: a Systematic Review." *Ophthalmology* 117, no. 1: 71–78.

Lee, E. Y., M. Y. Lee, S. W. Hong, et al. 2007. "Blockade of Oxidative Stress by Vitamin C Ameliorates Albuminuria and Renal Sclerosis in Experimental Diabetic Rats." *Yonsei Medical Journal* 48, no. 5: 847–55.

Lee, S. J., J. G. Kang, O. H. Ryu, et al. 2009. "Effects of Alpha-lipoic Acid on Transforming Growth Factor Beta1-p38 Mitogen-activated Protein Kinase-fibronectin Pathway in Diabetic Nephropathy." *Metabolism* 58, no. 5: 616–23.

Liepinsh, E., E. Skapare, E. Vavers, et al. 2012. "High L-carnitine Concentrations Do Not Prevent Late Diabetic Complications in Type 1 and 2 Diabetic Patients." *Nutrition Research* 32, no. 5: 320–27.

Ling, C., L. Groop, S. D. Guerra, et al. 2009. "Calpain-10 Expression Is Elevated in Pancreatic Islets from Patients with Type 2 Diabetes." *PLoS One* 4, no. 8: e6558.

Liu, F., Y. Zhang, M. Yang, et al. 2007. "Curative Effect of Alpha-lipoic Acid on Peripheral Neuropathy in Type 2 Diabetes: a Clinical Study." *Zhonghua Yi Xue Za Zhi* 87: 2706–09.

Liu, H. Y., S. Y. Cao, T. Hong, et al. 2009. "Insulin Is a Stronger Inducer of Insulin Resistance than Hyperglycemia in Mice with Type 1 Diabetes Mellitus (T1DM)." *Journal of Biolological Chemistry* 284: 27090–100.

Lodovici, M., E. Bigagli, G. Bardini, et al. 2009. "Lipoperoxidation and Antioxidant Capacity in Patients with Poorly Controlled Type 2 Diabetes." *Toxicology Industrial Health* 25, no. 4–5: 337–41.

Lu, Z., Q. Jia, R. Wang, et al. 2011. "Hypoglycemic Activities of A- and B-type Procyanidin Oligomer-rich Extracts from Different Cinnamon Barks." *Phytomedicine* 18, no. 4: 298–302.

Maalouf, R. M., A. A. Eid, Y. C. Gorin, et al. 2012. "Nox4-derived Reactive Oxygen Species Mediate Cardiomyocyte Injury in Early Type 1 Diabetes." *American Journal of Physiology—Cell Physiology* 302, no. 3: C597–604.

Malaguarnera, M., M. Vacante, T. Avitabile, et al. 2009. "L-Carnitine Supplementation Reduces Oxidized LDL Cholesterol in Patients with Diabetes." *American Journal of Clinical Nutrition* 89, no. 1: 71–76.

Malik, T. H., A. Cortini, D. Carassiti, et al. 2010. "The Alternative Pathway Is Critical for Pathogenic Complement Activation in Endotoxin- and Diet-induced Atherosclerosis in Low-density Lipoprotein Receptor-deficient Mice." *Circulation* 122, no. 19: 1948–56.

Malone, J. I., D. D. Cuthbertson, M. A. Malone, et al. 2006. "Cardio-protective Effects of Carnitine in Streptozotocin-induced Diabetic Rats." *Cardiovascular and Diabetology* 5:2.

Manolescu, D. C., A. Sima, and P. V. Bhat. 2010. "All-trans Retinoic Acid Lowers Serum Retinol-binding Protein 4 Concentrations and Increases Insulin Sensitivity in Diabetic Mice." *Journal of Nutrition* 140, no. 2: 311–16.

Mariappan, N., C. M. Elks, S. Sriramula, et al. 2010. "NF-kappa B-induced Oxidative Stress Contributes to Mitochondrial and Cardiac Dysfunction in Type II Diabetes." *Cardiovascular Research* 85: 473–83.

Martha, S., K. R. Devarakonda, R. N. Anreddy, et al. 2009. "Effect of Aspirin Treatment in Streptozotocin-induced Type 2 Diabetic Rats." *Methods and Findings in Experimental and Clinical Pharmacology* 31, no. 5: 331–35.

Martin-Gallan, P., A. Carrascosa, M. Gussinye, et al. 2003. "Biomarkers of

Diabetes-associated Oxidative Stress and Antioxidant Status in Young Diabetic Patients with or without Subclinical Complications." *Free Radicals Biolology and Medicine* 34, no. 12: 1563–74.

Masha, A., L. Brocato, S. Dinatale, et al. 2009. "N-acetylcysteine Is Able to Reduce the Oxidation Status and the Endothelial Activation after a High-glucose Content Meal in Patients with Type 2 Diabetes Mellitus." *Journal of Endocrinology Investigation* 32, no. 4: 352–56.

Mathieu, C., C. Gysemans, A. Giulietti, et al. 2005. "Vitamin D and Diabetes." *Diabetologia* 48, no. 7: 1247–57.

Matteucci, E., and O. Giampietro. 2000. "Oxidative Stress in Families of Type 1 Diabetic Patients." *Diabetes Care* 23, no. 8: 1182–86.

McCance, D. R., V. A. Holmes, M. J. Maresh, et al. 2010. "Vitamins C and E for Prevention of Pre-eclampsia in Women with Type 1 Diabetes (DAPIT): a Randomised Placebo-controlled Trial." *Lancet* 376, no. 9737: 259–66.

Mellor, K. M., R. H. Ritchie, and L. M. Delbridge. 2010. "Reactive Oxygen Species and Insulin Resistant Cardiomyopathy." *Clinical Experimental Pharmacology Physiology* 37: 222–28.

Minamino, T., M. Orimo, I. Shimizu, et al. 2009. "A Crucial Role for Adipose Tissue P53 in the Regulation of Insulin Resistance." *National Medicine* 15, no. 9: 1082–87.

Mingrone, G. 2004. "Carnitine in Type 2 Diabetes." *Annals of New York Academy of Sciences* 1033: 99–107.

Mishra, M., H. Kumar, S. Bajpai, et al. 2011. "Level of Serum IL-12 and Its Correlation with Endothelial Dysfunction, Insulin Resistance, Proinflammatory Cytokines and Lipid Profile in Newly Diagnosed Type 2 Diabetes." *Diabetes Research and Clinical Practice* 94, no. 2: 255–61.

Mitrovic, M., T. Ilic, E. Stokic, et al. 2011. "Influence of Glucoregulation Quality on C-reactive Protein, Interleukin-6 and Tumor Necrosis Factor-alpha Level in Patients with Diabetes Type 1." *Vojnosanitetski Pregled Military-medical and Pharmaceutical Review* 68, no. 9: 756–61.

Miyata, S., T. Miyata, A. Kada, et al. 2008. "[Aspirin Resistance]." *Brain Nerve* 60, no. 11: 1357–64.

Molfino, A., A. Cascino, C. Conte, et al. 2010. "Caloric Restriction and L-carnitine Administration Improves Insulin Sensitivity in Patients with Impaired Glucose Metabolism." *Journal of Parenteral and Enteral Nutrition* 34, no. 3: 295–99.

Mollo, R., F. Zaccardi, G. Scalone, et al. 2012. "Effect of Alpha-lipoic Acid on Platelet Reactivity in Type 1 Diabetic Patients." *Diabetes Care* 35, no. 2: 196–97.

Morales-Indiano, C., R. Lauzurica, M. C. Pastor, et al. 2009. "Greater Post-transplant Inflammation and Oxidation Are Associated with Worsening Kidney Function in Patients with Pretransplant Diabetes Mellitus." *Transplantation Proceedings* 41, no. 6: 2126–28.

Muellenbach, E. A., C. J. Diehl, M. K. Teachey, et al. 2008. "Interactions of the Advanced Glycation End Product Inhibitor Pyridoxamine and the Antioxidant Alpha-lipoic Acid on Insulin Resistance in the Obese Zucker Rat." *Metabolism* 57, no. 10: 1465–72.

Mustad, V. A., S. Demichele, Y. S. Huang, et al. 2006. "Differential Effects of N-3 Polyunsaturated Fatty Acids on Metabolic Control and Vascular Reactivity in the Type 2 Diabetic Ob/Ob Mouse." *Metabolism* 55, no. 10: 1365–74.

Nakhoul, F. M., R. Miller-Lotan, H. Awad, et al. 2009. "Pharmacogenomic Effect of Vitamin E on Kidney Structure and Function in Transgenic Mice with the Haptoglobin 2-2 Genotype and Diabetes Mellitus." *American Journal of Physiology and Renal Physiology* 296, no. 4: F830–38.

Naziroglu, M., N. Dilsiz, and M. Cay. 1999. "Protective Role of Intraperitoneally Administered Vitamins C and E and Selenium on the Levels of Lipid Peroxidation in the Lens of Rats Made Diabetic with Streptozotocin." *Biological Trace Element Research* 70, no. 3: 223–32.

Nebbioso, M., M. Federici, D. Rusciano, et al. 2012. "Oxidative Stress in Preretinopathic Diabetes Subjects and Antioxidants." *Diabetes Technology & Therapeutics* 14, no. 3: 257–63.

Neri, S., S. S. Signorelli, B. Torrisi, et al. 2005. "Effects of Antioxidant Supplementation on Postprandial Oxidative Stress and Endothelial Dysfunction: a Single-blind, 15-day Clinical Trial in Patients with Untreated Type 2 Diabetes, Subjects with Impaired Glucose Tolerance, and Healthy Controls." *Clinical Therapy* 27, no. 11: 1764–73.

Norris, J. M., X. Yin, M. M. Lamb, et al. 2007. "Omega-3 Polyunsaturated Fatty Acid Intake and Islet Autoimmunity in Children at Increased Risk for Type 1 Diabetes." *Journal of American Medical Association* 298, no. 12: 1420–28.

Nwosu, B. U., Z. G. Stavre, L. Maranda, et al. 2012. "Hepatic Dysfunction Is Associated with Vitamin D Deficiency and Poor Glycemic Control in

Diabetes Mellitus." *Journal of Pediatric Endocrinology & Metabolism* 25, no. 1–2: 181–86.

Odermarsky, M., J. Lykkesfeldt, and P. Liuba. 2009. "Poor Vitamin C Status Is Associated with Increased Carotid Intima-media Thickness, Decreased Microvascular Function, and Delayed Myocardial Repolarization in Young Patients with Type 1 Diabetes." *American Journal of Clinical Nutrition* 90, no. 2: 447–52.

Ogawa, H., M. Nakayama, T. Morimoto, et al. 2008. "Low-dose Aspirin for Primary Prevention of Atherosclerotic Events in Patients with Type 2 Diabetes: a Randomized Controlled Trial." *Journal of American Medical Association* 300, no. 18: 2134–41.

Onat, A., G. Hergenc, G. Can, et al. 2010. "Serum Complement C3: a Determinant of Cardiometabolic Risk, Additive to the Metabolic Syndrome, in Middle-aged Population." *Metabolism: Clinical and Experimental* 59, no. 5: 628–34.

Ortis, F., P. Pirot, N. Naamane, et al. 2008. "Induction of Nuclear Factor-kappaB and Its Downstream Genes by TNF-alpha and IL-1beta Has a Pro-apoptotic Role in Pancreatic Beta Cells." *Diabetologia* 51, no. 7: 1213–25.

Osorio, J. M., C. Ferreyra, A. Perez, et al. 2009. "Prediabetic States, Subclinical Atheromatosis, and Oxidative Stress in Renal Transplant Patients." *Transplantation Proceedings* 41, no. 6: 2148–50.

Owu, D. U., A. O. Obembe, C. R. Nwokocha, et al. 2012. "Gastric Ulceration in Diabetes Mellitus: Protective Role of Vitamin C." *ISRN Gastroenterology*, doi:10.5402/2012/362805.

Ozgen, I. T., M. E. Tascilar, P. Bilir, et al. 2012. "Oxidative Stress in Obese Children and Its Relation with Insulin Resistance." *Journal of Pediatric Endocrinology and Metabolism* 25, no. 3–4: 261–66.

Ozkaya, D., M. Naziroglu, A. Armagan, et al. 2011. "Dietary Vitamin C and E Modulates Oxidative Stress Induced-kidney and Lens Injury in Diabetic Aged Male Rats through Modulating Glucose Homeostasis and Antioxidant Systems." *Cell Biochemistry and Function* 29, no. 4: 287–93.

Padmalayam, I., S. Hasham, U. Saxena, et al. 2009. "Lipoic Acid Synthase (LASY): a Novel Role in Inflammation, Mitochondrial Function, and Insulin Resistance." *Diabetes* 58, no. 3: 600–608.

Palomer, X., J. M. Gonzalez-Clemente, F. Blanco-Vaca, et al. 2008. "Role of Vitamin D in the Pathogenesis of Type 2 Diabetes Mellitus." *Diabetes, Obesity and Metabolism* 10, no. 3: 185–97.

Park, N. Y., S. K. Park, and Y. Lim. 2011. "Long-term Dietary Antioxidant Cocktail Supplementation Effectively Reduces Renal Inflammation in Diabetic Mice." *The British Journal of Nutrition* 106, no. 10: 1514–21.

Patel, C., H. Ghanim, S. Ravishankar, et al. 2007. "Prolonged Reactive Oxygen Species Generation and Nuclear Factor-kappaB Activation after a High-fat, High-carbohydrate Meal in the Obese." *Journal of Clinical Endocrinology and Metabolism* 92, no. 11: 4476–79.

Patel, D., and M. Moonis. 2007. "Clinical Implications of Aspirin Resistance." *Expert Review of Cardiovascular Therapy* 5, no. 5: 969–75.

Patumraj, S., N. Wongeakin, P. Sridulyakul, et al. 2006. "Combined Effects of Curcumin and Vitamin C to Protect Endothelial Dysfunction in the Iris Tissue of STZ-induced Diabetic Rats." *Clinical Hemorheology and Microcirculation* 35, no. 4: 481–89.

Peuchant, E., J. L. Brun, V. Rigalleau, et al. 2004. "Oxidative and Antioxidative Status in Pregnant Women with Either Gestational or Type 1 Diabetes." *Clinical Biochemistry* 37, no. 4: 293–98.

Pietropaoli, D., A. Monaco, R. Del Pinto, et al. 2012. "Advanced Glycation End Products: Possible Link between Metabolic Syndrome and Periodontal Diseases." *International Journal of Immunopathology and Pharmacology* 25, no. 1: 9–17.

Pitocco, D., E. Di Stasio, F. Romitelli, et al. 2008. "Hypouricemia Linked to an Overproduction of Nitric Oxide Is an Early Marker of Oxidative Stress in Female Subjects with Type 1 Diabetes." *Diabetes/Metabolism Research and Reviews* 24, no. 4: 318–23.

Pittas, A. G., J. Nelson, J. Mitri, et al. 2012. "Plasma 25-hydroxyvitamin D and Progression to Diabetes in Patients at Risk for Diabetes: an Ancillary Analysis in the Diabetes Prevention Program." *Diabetes Care* 35, no. 3: 565–73.

Poh, Z. X., and K. P. Goh. 2009. "A Current Update on the Use of Alpha Lipoic Acid in the Management of Type 2 Diabetes Mellitus." *Endocrine, Metabolic and Immune Disorders—Drug Targets* 9: 392–98.

Poorabbas, A., F. Fallah, J. Bagdadchi, et al. 2007. "Determination of Free L-carnitine Levels in Type II Diabetic Women with and without Complications." *European Journal of Clinical Nutrition* 61, no. 7: 892–95.

Pooya, S., M. D. Jalali, A. D. Jazayery, et al. 2009. "The Efficacy of Omega-3 Fatty Acid Supplementation on Plasma Homocysteine and

Malondialdehyde Levels of Type 2 Diabetic Patients." *Nutrition Metabolism and Cardiovascular Disease* 20: 326–31.

Power, R. A., M. W. Hulver, J. Y. Zhang, et al. 2007. "Carnitine Revisited: Potential Use as Adjunctive Treatment in Diabetes." *Diabetologia* 50, no. 4: 824–32.

Pradhan, A. D., N. R. Cook, J. E. Manson, et al. 2009. "A Randomized Trial of Low-dose Aspirin in the Prevention of Clinical Type 2 Diabetes in Women." *Diabetes Care* 32, no. 1: 3–8.

Prasad, K. N. 2011. *Micronutrients in Health and Disease.* Boca Raton, Florida: CRC Press.

Prasad, K. N., B. Kumar, X. D. Yan, et al. 2003. "Alpha-tocopheryl Succinate, the Most Effective Form of Vitamin E for Adjuvant Cancer Treatment: a Review." *Journal of American College of Nutrition* 22, no. 2: 108–17.

Prasad, K. N., and K. C. Prasad. 2011. *Fighting Cancer with Vitamins and Antioxidants.* Rochester, Vermont: Healing Arts Press.

Price, H. C., and R. R. Holman. 2009. "Primary Prevention of Cardiovascular Events in Diabetes: Is There a Role for Aspirin?" *Nature Clinical Practice Cardiovascular Medicine* 6, no. 3: 168–69.

Rajasekar, P., and C. V. Anuradha. 2007. "L-Carnitine Inhibits Protein Glycation in Vitro and in Vivo: Evidence for a Role in Diabetic Management." *Acta Diabetologica* 44, no. 2: 83–90.

Rasheed, Z., H. A. Al-Shobaili, A. A. Alzolibani, et al. 2011. "Immunological Functions of Oxidized Human Immunoglobulin G in Type 1 Diabetes Mellitus: Its Potential Role in Diabetic Smokers as a Biomarker of Elevated Oxidative Stress." *Disease Markers* 31, no. 1: 47–54.

Reny, J. L., R. F. Bonvini, I. Barazer, et al. 2009. "The Concept of Aspirin 'Resistance': Mechanisms and Clinical Relevance." *La Revue de Medecine Interne [Review of Internal Medicine]* 30: 1020–29.

Rizzo, M. R., A. M. Abbatecola, M. Barbieri, et al. 2008. "Evidence for Anti-inflammatory Effects of Combined Administration of Vitamin E and C in Older Persons with Impaired Fasting Glucose: Impact on Insulin Action." *Journal of American College of Nutrition* 27, no. 4: 505–11.

Ruggenenti, P., D. Cattaneo, G. Loriga, et al. 2009. "Ameliorating Hypertension and Insulin Resistance in Subjects at Increased Cardiovascular Risk: Effects of Acetyl-L-carnitine Therapy." *Hypertension* 54, no. 3: 567–74.

Sacco, M., F. Pellegrini, M. C. Roncaglioni, et al. 2003. "Primary Prevention of Cardiovascular Events with Low-dose Aspirin and Vitamin E in Type 2 Diabetic Patients: Results of the Primary Prevention Project (PPP) Trial." *Diabetes Care* 26, no. 12: 3264–72.

Samocha-Bonet, D., L. V. Campbell, T. A. Mori, et al. 2012. "Overfeeding Reduces Insulin Sensitivity and Increases Oxidative Stress, without Altering Markers of Mitochondrial Content and Function in Humans." *PloS One* 7, no. 5: e36320.

Sankhla, M., T. K. Sharma, K. Mathur, et al. 2012. "Relationship of Oxidative Stress with Obesity and Its Role in Obesity Induced Metabolic Syndrome." *Clinical Laboratory* 58, no. 5–6: 385–92.

Sasaki, J., T. Miwa, and M. Odawara. 2012. "Administration of Highly Purified Eicosapentaenoic Acid to Statin-treated Diabetic Patients Further Improves Vascular Function." *Endocrine Journal* 59, no. 4: 297–304.

Sedeek, M., G. Callera, A. Montezano, et al. 2010. "Critical Role of Nox4-based NADPH Oxidase in Glucose-induced Oxidative Stress in the Kidney: Implications in Type 2 Diabetic Nephropathy." *American Journal of Physiology Renal Physiology* 299, no. 6: F1348–58.

Shankar, S. S., B. Mirzamohammadi, J. P. Walsh, et al. 2004. "L-carnitine May Attenuate Free Fatty Acid-induced Endothelial Dysfunction." *Annals of New York Academy of Sciences* 1033: 189–97.

Sharma, S., R. P. Agrawal, M. Choudhary, et al. 2011. "Beneficial Effect of Chromium Supplementation on Glucose, HbA1C and Lipid Variables in Individuals with Newly Onset Type-2 Diabetes." *Journal of Trace Element in Medicine and Biology* 25, no. 3: 149–53.

Sima, A. A. 2007. "Acetyl-L-carnitine in Diabetic Polyneuropathy: Experimental and Clinical Data." *CNS Drugs* 21, suppl 1: 13–23.

Singh, U., and I. Jialal. 2008. "Alpha-lipoic Acid Supplementation and Diabetes." *Nutrition Review* 66, no. 11: 646–57.

Sohet, F. M., A. M. Neyrinck, B. D. Pachikian, et al. 2009. "Coenzyme Q10 Supplementation Lowers Hepatic Oxidative Stress and Inflammation Associated with Diet-induced Obesity in Mice." *Biochemical Pharmacology* 78: 1391–1400.

Sokmen, B., H. Basaraner, and R. Yanardag. 2012. "Combined Effects of Treatment with Vitamin C, Vitamin E and Selenium on the Skin of Diabetic Rats." *Human & Experimental Toxicology* 32, no. 4: 379–84.

Solfrizzi, V., C. Capurso, A. M. Colacicco, et al. 2006. "Efficacy and Tolerability of Combined Treatment with L-carnitine and Simvastatin in Lowering Lipoprotein(a) Serum Levels in Patients with Type 2 Diabetes Mellitus." *Atherosclerosis* 188, no. 2: 455–61.

Soneru, I. L., T. Khan, Z. Orfalian, et al. 1997. "Acetyl-L-carnitine Effects on Nerve Conduction and Glycemic Regulation in Experimental Diabetes." *Endocrine Research* 23, no. 1–2: 27–36.

Song, F., W. Jia, Y. Yao, et al. 2007. "Oxidative Stress, Antioxidant Status and DNA Damage in Patients with Impaired Glucose Regulation and Newly Diagnosed Type 2 Diabetes." *Clinical Sciences* 112, no. 12: 599–606.

Song, Y., N. R. Cook, C. M. Albert, et al. 2009a. "Effects of Vitamins C and E and Beta-carotene on the Risk of Type 2 Diabetes in Women at High Risk of Cardiovascular Disease: a Randomized Controlled Trial." *American Journal of Clinical Nutrition* 90, no. 2: 429–37.

Song, Y., N. R. Cook, C. M. Albert, et al. 2009b. "Effect of Homocysteine-lowering Treatment with Folic Acid and B Vitamins on Risk of Type 2 Diabetes in Women: a Randomized, Controlled Trial." *Diabetes* 58, no. 8:1921–28.

Song, Y., Q. Xu, Y. Park, et al. 2011. "Multivitamins, Individual Vitamin and Mineral Supplements, and Risk of Diabetes among Older U.S. Adults." *Diabetes Care* 34, no. 1: 108–14.

Sridulyakul, P., D. Chakraphan, and S. Patumraj. 2006. "Vitamin C Supplementation Could Reverse Diabetes-induced Endothelial Cell Dysfunction in Mesenteric Microcirculation in STZ-rats." *Clinical Hemorheology in Microcirculation* 34, 1–2: 315–21.

Stirban, A., S. Nandrean, C. Gotting, et al. 2010. "Effects of N-3 Fatty Acids on Macro- and Microvascular Function in Subjects with Type 2 Diabetes Mellitus." *American Journal of Clinical Nutrition* 91, no. 3: 808–13.

Su, Y. X., J. Hong, Q. Yan, et al. 2010. "Increased Serum Retinol-binding Protein-4 Levels in Pregnant Women with and without Gestational Diabetes Mellitus." *Diabetes & Metabolism* 36, no. 6, part 1: 470–75.

Sugimura, Y., T. Murase, K. Kobayashi, et al. 2009. "Alpha-lipoic Acid Reduces Congenital Malformations in the Offspring of Diabetic Mice." *Diabetes/Metabolism Research and Review* 25, no. 3: 287–94.

Suksomboon, N., N. Poolsup, S. Boonkaew, et al. 2011. "Meta-analysis of the Effect of Herbal Supplement on Glycemic Control in Type 2 Diabetes." *Journal of Ethnopharmacology* 137, no. 3: 1328–33.

Suzuki, S., Y. Hinokio, M. Ohtomo, et al. 1998. "The Effects of Coenzyme Q10 Treatment on Maternally Inherited Diabetes Mellitus and Deafness, and Mitochondrial DNA 3243 (A to G) Mutation." *Diabetologia* 41, no. 5: 584–88.

Tankova, T., D. Koev, and L. Dakovska. 2004. "Alpha-lipoic Acid in the Treatment of Autonomic Diabetic Neuropathy (Controlled, Randomized, Open-label Study)." *Romanian Journal of Internal Medicine* 42, no. 2: 457–64.

Tepper, B. J., Y. K. Kim, V. Shete, et al. 2010. "Serum Retinol-binding Protein 4 (RBP4) and Retinol in a Cohort of Borderline Obese Women with and without Gestational Diabetes." *Clinical Biochemistry* 43, no. 3: 320–23.

Tessier, D. M., A. Khalil, L. Trottier, et al. 2009. "Effects of Vitamin C Supplementation on Antioxidants and Lipid Peroxidation Markers in Elderly Subjects with Type 2 Diabetes." *Archives of Gerontology and Geriatrics* 48, no. 1: 67–72.

Todoric, J., M. Loffler, J. Huber, et al. 2006. "Adipose Tissue Inflammation Induced by High-fat Diet in Obese Diabetic Mice Is Prevented by N-3 Polyunsaturated Fatty Acids." *Diabetologia* 49, no. 9: 2109–19.

Troseid, M., I. Seljeflot, E. M. Hjerkinn, et al. 2009. "Interleukin-18 Is a Strong Predictor of Cardiovascular Events in Elderly Men with the Metabolic Syndrome: Synergistic Effect of Inflammation and Hyperglycemia." *Diabetes Care* 32, no. 3: 486–92.

Tsai, G. Y., J. Z. Cui, H. Syed, et al. 2009. "Effect of N-acetylcysteine on the Early Expression of Inflammatory Markers in the Retina and Plasma of Diabetic Rats." *Clinical and Experimental Ophthalmology* 37, no. 2: 223–31.

Tsuneki, H., N. Sekizaki, T. Suzuki, et al. 2007. "Coenzyme Q10 Prevents High Glucose-induced Oxidative Stress in Human Umbilical Vein Endothelial Cells." *European Journal of Pharmacology* 566, no. 1–3: 1–10.

Ulusu, N. N., M. Sahilli, A. Avci, et al. 2003. "Pentose Phosphate Pathway, Glutathione-dependent Enzymes and Antioxidant Defense during Oxidative Stress in Diabetic Rodent Brain and Peripheral Organs: Effects of Stobadine and Vitamin E." *Neurochemical Research* 28, no. 6: 815–23.

van Oostrom, O., D. P. de Kleijn, J. O. Fledderus, et al. 2009. "Folic Acid Supplementation Normalizes the Endothelial Progenitor Cell Transcriptome of Patients with Type 1 Diabetes: a Case-control Pilot Study." *Cardiovascular Diabetology* 8: 47.

Venturini, D., A. N. Simao, N. A. Scripes, et al. 2012. "Evaluation of Oxidative Stress in Overweight Subjects with or without Metabolic Syndrome." *Obesity* 20, no 12: 2361–66.

Villegas, R., Y. B. Xiang, T. Elasy, et al. 2011. "Fish, Shellfish, and Long-chain N-3 Fatty Acid Consumption and Risk of Incident Type 2 Diabetes in Middle-aged Chinese Men and Women." *American Journal of Clinical Nutrition* 94, no. 2: 543–51.

Wang, T., F. H. Fu, B. Han, et al. 2009. "Aspirin Attenuates Cerebral Ischemic Injury in Diabetic Rats." *Experimental and Clinical Endocrinology & Diabetes* 117, no. 4: 181–85.

Wang, Z. Q., and W. T. Cefalu. 2010. "Current Concepts about Chromium Supplementation in Type 2 Diabetes and Insulin Resistance." *Current Diabetes Reports* 10, no. 2: 145–51.

Wong, C. Y., K. H. Yiu, S. W. Li, et al. 2010. "Fish-oil Supplement Has Neutral Effects on Vascular and Metabolic Function but Improves Renal Function in Patients with Type 2 Diabetes Mellitus." *Diabetic Medicine: a Journal of the British Diabetic Association* 27, no. 1: 54–60.

Wu, J. H., R. Micha, F. Imamura, et al. 2012. "Omega-3 Fatty Acids and Incident Type 2 Diabetes: a Systematic Review and Meta-analysis." *The British Journal of Nutrition* 107, suppl 2: S214–27.

Xia, Z., Z. Guo, P. R. Nagareddy, et al. 2006. "Antioxidant N-acetylcysteine Restores Myocardial Mn-SOD Activity and Attenuates Myocardial Dysfunction in Diabetic Rats." *European Journal of Pharmacology* 544, no. 1–3: 118–25.

Xia, Z., K. H. Kuo, P. R. Nagareddy, et al. 2007. "N-acetylcysteine Attenuates PKCbeta2 Overexpression and Myocardial Hypertrophy in Streptozotocin-induced Diabetic Rats." *Cardiovascular Research* 73, no. 4: 770–82.

Yang, J., Y. Park, H. Zhang, et al. 2009. "Feed-forward Signaling of TNF-alpha and NF-kappaB via IKK-beta Pathway Contributes to Insulin Resistance and Coronary Arteriolar Dysfunction in Type 2 Diabetic Mice." *American Journal of Physiology—Heart and Circulation Physiology* 296, no. 6: H1850–58.

Yessoufou, A., N. Soulaimann, S. A. Merzouk, et al. 2006. "N-3 Fatty Acids Modulate Antioxidant Status in Diabetic Rats and Their Macrosomic Offspring." *International Journal of Obesity* 30, no. 5: 739–50.

Yokota, T., S. Kinugawa, K. Hirabayashi, et al. 2009. "Oxidative Stress in

Skeletal Muscle Impairs Mitochondrial Respiration and Limits Exercise Capacity in Type 2 Diabetic Mice." *American Journal of Physiology—Heart and Circulation Physiology* 297, no. 3: H1069–77.

Young, J. M., C. M. Florkowski, S. L. Molyneux, et al. 2012. "A Randomized, Double-blind, Placebo-controlled Crossover Study of Coenzyme Q10 Therapy in Hypertensive Patients with the Metabolic Syndrome." *American Journal of Hypertension* 25, no. 2: 261–70.

Younis, N., S. Williams, and H. Soran. 2009. "Aspirin Therapy and Primary Prevention of Cardiovascular Disease in Diabetes Mellitus." *Diabetes, Obesity and Metabolism* 11: 997–1000.

Zhang, Y., P. Han, N. Wu, et al. 2011. "Amelioration of Lipid Abnormalities by Alpha-lipoic Acid through Antioxidative and Anti-inflammatory Effects." *Obesity* (Silver Spring, Md.) 19, no. 8: 1647–53.

Zhou, S. J., L. Yelland, A. J. McPhee, et al. 2012. "Fish-oil Supplementation in Pregnancy Does Not Reduce the Risk of Gestational Diabetes or Preeclampsia." *American Journal of Clinical Nutrition* 95, no. 6: 1378–84.

Ziegler, D., A. Ametov, A. Barinov, et al. 2006. "Oral Treatment with Alpha-lipoic Acid Improves Symptomatic Diabetic Polyneuropathy: the SYDNEY 2 Trial." *Diabetes Care* 29, no. 11: 2365–70.

Ziegler, D., P. A. Low, W. J. Litchy, et al. 2011. "Efficacy and Safety of Antioxidant Treatment with Alpha-lipoic Acid over 4 Years in Diabetic Polyneuropathy: the NATHAN 1 Trial." *Diabetes Care* 34, no. 9: 2054–60.

Zunino, S. J., D. H. Storms, and C. B. Stephensen. 2007. "Diets Rich in Polyphenols and Vitamin A Inhibit the Development of Type I Autoimmune Diabetes in Nonobese Diabetic Mice." *Journal of Nutrition* 137, no. 5: 1216–21.

About the Author

Kedar N. Prasad, Ph.D., former president of the International Society for Nutrition and Cancer, obtained a master's degree in zoology from the University of Bihar, Ranchi, India, and his Ph.D. degree in radiation biology from the University of Iowa, Iowa City, in 1963. He then attended the Brookhaven National Laboratory on Long Island for postdoctoral training before joining the Department of Radiology at the University of Colorado Health Sciences Center, where he became a professor in 1980. Later, he was appointed director of the Center for Vitamins and Cancer Research at the University of Colorado School of Medicine. In 1982, he was invited by the Nobel Prize Committee to nominate a candidate for the Nobel Prize in medicine, and in 1999 he was selected to deliver the Harold Harper Lecture at the meeting of the American College of Advancement in Medicine.

His published papers and articles have appeared in such illustrious publications as *Science, Nature,* and *Proceedings of the National Academy of Sciences of the United States of America* (PNAS). He is also the author of several book chapters and eighteen books, including *Fighting Cancer with Vitamins and Antioxidants.* A member of several professional organizations, he serves as an ad-hoc member of various study sections of the National Institutes of Health (NIH) and has consistently obtained NIH grants for his research.

Kedar N. Prasad is frequently an invited speaker at national and international meetings on nutrition and cancer. He began researching various types of cancers and the effects of radiation on human tissues in 1963. Over the next twenty-five years, he continued his biological research at five major universities and research labs, studying the relationships between micronutrients, cancer, and radiation and focusing on the effects that micronutrients have on human cells and the manner in which they interact with mainstream medical therapies for many common diseases. He found that certain combinations of micronutrients when taken in conjunction with standard treatments, such as chemotherapy, enhanced and complemented the effects of these traditional therapies. The findings inspired him to further his research to determine the effects that these micronutrient combinations might have on other diseases and on general human health.

His present research interests are in the areas of radiation protection, nutrition and cancer, and nutrition and neurological diseases, particularly Alzheimer's disease and Parkinson's disease. Since 2005 he has been the chief scientific officer of the Premier Micronutrient Corporation, which produces antioxidant micronutrient formulations to fight disease and promote a healthy lifestyle.

Index

216